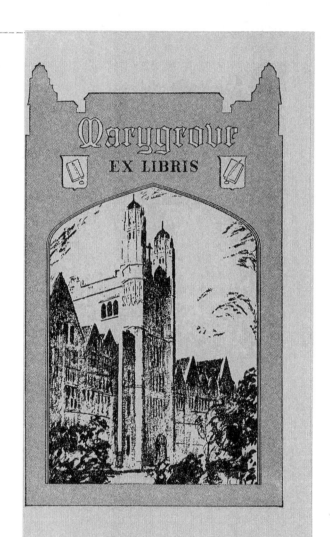

HEROIC SANCTITY
AND
INSANITY

HEROIC SANCTITY

AND

INSANITY

An Introduction to the
Spiritual Life and Mental Hygiene

By

THOMAS VERNER MOORE, Carthusian
(In Religion, Pablo Maria)

Formerly Head of the Department of Psychology and Psychiatry and Director of the Child Guidance Center at the Catholic University of America, Washington, D.C.

GRUNE & STRATTON — 1959 — New York and London

Dedicated
to
Sister Genevieve of the Holy Face*
and of
St. Thérèse
Céline
The Surviving Sister
of the
Little Flower

*Sister Genevieve died while this work was in press.

O Verbum aeternum
Accipere digneris munus hujus opusculi
Quod Tibi humiliter offerre praesumo
In spiritu reparationis
Et in honorem sponsae Tuae parvulae
Sanctae Theresiae a Jesu Infante
et
A Sancto Vultu

CONTENTS

Preface

Heroic Sanctity and Insanity appears at a time when psychiatrists are giving special attention to the relation between religion and psychiatry. But so far the important distinction has not been made between those whose names are on a baptismal register and those who are heroic in their fidelity to the commandments of God, given in the Old Law and to the invitation of Christ in which those commandments find their complete expression in the New Law.

Few psychiatrists in our day could, without any special study, sit down and write out a detailed description of just what heroic sanctity means.

The present book points out in the beginning that Christ asks all men to strive for heroic sanctity and then goes on to show[1] how this means that in heroic sanctity there can be no vice. Some virtues must be practiced in an heroic degree, and all others that are possible for one to practice in his life must be present at least as outstanding accomplishments, that is in a high, but not necessarily heroic, degree.

The work then goes on to a short introduction to psychiatry, stressing those mental disorders that have their roots in our mental life. The attempt is made to make all this clear and also easy reading by numerous interesting examples. From this discussion it appears that there are a number of ways in which *great* sanctity may strengthen the personality so that instead of a mental breakdown we have a vigorous character bobbing up serenely at his daily duties. Sanctity is most important in *preventing* mental breakdowns; but a reform of the moral and spiritual life can sometimes be an important factor in *therapy*. This does not imply by any means that one can always or ever generally dispense with the services of a psychiatrist.

Extensive use is made of the development of the sanctity of St. Thérèse of Lisieux. A psychiatric study of the growth of her personality shows that it was a normal, continuous process of unfolding from about two years of age until her death. What has been called a mental breakdown in her eleventh year turns out on investigation to have been a delirium such as often accompanies various infectious diseases of childhood. She suffered bitterly from the death of her mother when she was about four and a half; and from the parting with her two sisters, to enter Carmel,

---

[1] From the work of Benedict XIV, *On the Beatification and Canonization of Saints.*

ix

who had successively taken the part of a mother to her. But there was never anything like the abiding, total disorganization of her personality which would indicate a psychosis nor what Adolf Meyer termed "that part reaction which involves a disability beyond the powers of the patient to control, and creates a long lasting disability that seriously interferes with daily life."

The psychiatrist often has a very difficult problem to decide between (1) a major mental disorder (a psychosis), and (2) that "part reaction" which is termed a psychoneurosis, and (3) an emotional reaction to the stress and strain of life which is indeed severe but within the limits of normal fluctuations of mood. This work offers a study of these normal fluctuations of mood which may well be helpful to many.

In a communication to the *Catholic Herald*, London, June 13, 1958, an anonymous writer stated that he had, to the great surprise of his Catholic psychiatrist, demonstrated in himself that emotional maturity may be attained by a "sensible attitude." He expressed the hope for a Catholic writer who would "correlate the facts of mental hygiene with the full body of religious truth." The present work, while pointing out that *the whole of psychotherapy is by no means religious therapy*, maintains that religious ideals, lived out in a deep spiritual life, can and do prevent some mental disorders and at times relieve or even cure conditions in which all other forms of therapy, by themselves, are powerless.

For whom is this book intended? (a) For that vast number who at the present day are striving to attain spiritual perfection. The ideals of heroism in the various virtues, as formulated for the process of the canonization of saints, clarifies the atmosphere for those who want to live so as to attain to perfect sanctity.

(b) The author hopes that *Heroic Sanctity and Insanity* will help those on whom the stress and strain of life lies heavy, and enable them to keep the fluctuations of their emotional life within normal limits so that they will always be able to answer the call of duty.

There is an increasing attitude of sympathy between the clergy and psychiatrists toward religion. The clergy should have some knowledge of psychiatry and psychiatrists should at least know what religion is. Can true religion be presented without a clear outline of sanctity? Religion without sanctity is sounding brass and tinkling cymbal. Can you stage Hamlet and cut out the part of the Prince of Denmark?

THOMAS VERNER MOORE

I. The Heroic Virtue of the Saints

CHAPTER I

Heroic Sanctity and the Laity

ALL THE FAITHFUL CAN AND SHOULD TRY TO REACH SPIRITUAL PERFECTION

IS THERE ANY obligation upon a layman to strive for heroic sanctity? Or is the sanctity required of a layman on an essentially lower level than that demanded of priests and religious?

This does not mean: are the laity bound by the same obligation to strive for perfection as religious who are bound by vows? All men are bound to obey those placed over them in a position of authority, but there comes an added obligation when one vows obedience to his superiors.

When we examine the matter it seems theologically clear that all the faithful are called by God to the summit of Christian perfection. In Christianity there should be no second class Christians. This seems evident from Christ's own words to the common people gathered before Him while He was preaching the Sermon on the Mount: "Be you therefore perfect, as also your heavenly Father is perfect." (Matthew V:48). And when we look at what He urged just before these words, we see that He certainly meant a degree of perfection that is heroic and seldom found in daily life: Turn the other cheek to one who slaps your face, he who would take away your coat, let him have your cloak also. "Love your enemies, do good to them that hate you; and pray for them that persecute and calumniate you." (Matthew V:44).

And then Our Lord lays down the command, "Thou shalt love the Lord thy God with thy whole heart and with thy whole soul and with all thy strength and with all thy mind, and thy neighbor as thyself." (Luke X:27). One cannot interpret these words without admitting that they mean that we must love God as much as we possibly can; and take care of our neighbor in any great necessity even as we would take care of ourselves were we in his plight. As we shall see, the very essence of spiritual perfection is the love of God. This is measured not by emotional fervor but by deeds: what we will do and endure for the love of God.

And then there is Our Lord's last prayer at the first Eucharistic banquet. In this prayer each one of us is included, for He said "not for them only do I pray, but for them also who through their word shall believe in Me. That they all may be one, as Thou, Father in Me, and I in Thee—I in them and Thou in Me, that they may be made perfect in One." (John XVII:20, 21, 23).

All this implies a spiritual perfection in which the soul on earth is assimilated to the life of the Blessed Trinity. Now this was meant not for the Apostles alone, not for the bishops and priests alone who would follow after them, but for all the men, women and children who through the work of the Apostles would believe in Christ down through the centuries to the end of time.

But let us clarify what is here meant by pointing out that it is not necessary to be perfect in order to belong to the mystical body of the Church, for Pius VI condemned as heretical the concept that only those among the faithful belong to the mystical body of the Church who are perfect adorers in spirit and in truth.[1]

One will save his soul if he dies in the state of grace without having attained to spiritual perfection. One should interpret in the light of this the following words of Our Lord: "How narrow is the gate and straight the way that leadeth to life; and few there are that find it." (Matthew VII:14). It does not necessarily mean that few are saved, but rather that few answer Christ's call and set out on the way to perfection in this life.

In the year 816 there was held at Aix-la-Chapelle a council which discussed the ideals of the spiritual life for priests, nuns and, to some extent, for the laity. It interpreted the words "narrow gate and straight path" to refer to the road to spiritual perfection, and said: "Not only must monks and nuns, but also all included under the name of Christian, enter upon the straight and narrow path. . . . One must also realize that the more one humbles himself in this present life, for the love of Christ, the greater will be his happy reward in the life to come."[2] From this it is clear that in the early ninth century, priests,

---

[1] Pius VI, Bulla Auctorem fidei contra Ps. Synodum Pistorienem, cited in Josephus de Guibert Documenta Ecclesiastica Christianae Perfectionis, etc. Rome, 1931, Gregorian University, 516, p. 337.

[2] Quoted from Joseph de Guibert, op. cit., pp. 70, 117.

nuns, and the laity were looked upon as all called to strive for perfection.

Coming to our own days, Pius XI wrote as follows: "In a particular manner do we desire that you should call back the faithful to the duty that each one has to seek his own personal sanctity. For there are far too many who never think of eternal life or entirely neglect the salvation of their souls. Wherefore, venerable brothers, bring it about by the Salesian Institute that the people should understand that sanctity is not a rare favor granted to only a few, but the common lot and duty of all."[3]

And in 1930 the same Holy Father wrote: "All men of whatever condition, in whatever honorable walk of life they may be, can and ought to imitate that most perfect example of holiness placed before man by God, namely, Christ Jesus, Our Lord, and by God's grace to arrive at the *summit* of perfection."[4]

According to this it seems that we can maintain without fear of contradiction that Christ's teaching is expressed in the mind of the Church by the statement that all the faithful whether married or single *can and ought* to do all they can to arrive at the summit of Christian perfection.

2. The Essence of Perfection is the Love of God

One might conceive of spiritual perfection as sinlessness. Sin is a free transgression of the law of God. God's law is the manifestation of His Divine Will. When one sins he chooses what he himself wants and rejects what God wants. But when one obeys God's law he wills what God wills and gives up his own personal desire. But that is the best sign one can have that one loves God—fidelity to Him in the hour of temptation.

The more fully a creature attains the end for which it was created, the greater is its perfection. The highest possible end of an intellectual being is that he should know and obey the Infinite Truth, God, the Source of all that is.

Sin clouds the mind. Blessed are the clean of heart for they shall see God. This union of our will with the will of God is charity. For charity as an act is a free, responsible choice of that which is truly good. It is by doing the will of God that we become perfect.

[3] Encyclical Letter (Rerum Omnium) to the Society of St. Francis de Sales (Salesians) January 26, 1923. Cited from Guibert, op. cit., No. 639, p. 427. Italics mine.

[4] Pius XI, Encyclical on Christian Marriage (Casti Connubii) Dec. 31, 1930. National Catholic Welfare Edition, 1931, pp. 10-11. Italics mine.

"The perfection of Christian life consists fundamentally and essentially in charity manifesting itself mainly in the love of God and,
secondarily, in the love of our neighbor."[5]

3. The Ordinary Means of Attaining to Sanctity

If we have realized that all are called to the summit of Christian
perfection and recall that this is fully attained only in eternal life when
we shall be made like to God because we shall see Him as He is, it will
be clear to us that over and above our own puny efforts, we must have
supernatural, divine help.

This help is imparted to us through a Eucharistic life, for without
Christ we can do nothing. Devout souls, therefore, in pursuit of
perfection, often go daily to Mass and Holy Communion and to confession every week. No one can attain to perfection except with the
aid of Christ. In Russia and China, Holy Mass and confession are not
generally available to all. God will, however, make it possible that all
who truly seek Him, no matter where they may be, will find Him.
But in most countries of the world and in all larger towns, the sacraments are in general easily available and become to all who approach
them the most important means of their sanctification.

Besides the sacraments, the ordinary means of sanctification are
prayer, vocal and mental, holy reading and the practice of self-denial;
and in a particular manner the exact and loving fulfillment of the
duties of our state in life.

A recent writer having dwelt on the importance in family life of
proper housing, adequate play space for children, activities that have
to do with income and repairs, and the common needs of families,
suddenly stops and says: "At this point you may say, 'But where's the
spirituality?' More than likely you mean 'Where's the monasticism?'—
such as group prayer, extraordinary asceticism and new forms of
worship?"[6]

One must remember that both religious and laity are called by
Christ to the very summit of Christian perfection, and that the means
to attain it are essentially the same: the sacraments, vocal and mental
prayer, holy reading and the practice of self-denial. The differences

---

[5] St. Thomas *Summa Theologica*, 2.2. Q. CLXXXIV, iii.

[6] Ed Willock, "Spirituality and Lay Community" in *Spiritual Life*, 1958, 4, p. 136.
One can only regret a tendency in this article to develop a rift between the clergy
and the faithful.

between the use of these means by monks and members of the laity is only accidental.

As to group prayer, it is a sound principle that every social unit should have some form of group prayer so that it may serve God as a unit, not as a number of isolated individuals. Group prayer at meals goes back to the earliest days of Christianity.[7] St. Ignatius of Antioch wrote to the Trallians: "Persevere in your concord and in your community prayers."[8]

Some fifty years ago, other than Grace before and after meals, anything like group prayer in the families of our country was the exception rather than the rule. But in recent years the family rosary has become the common, if not the usual, practice in Catholic families. Furthermore, in many regions, Catholic families living near each other are linked together, one visiting another alternately for what might be termed the interfamily rosary. It is a practice which increases greatly that mutual charity which should abound between all the faithful.

Then the liturgy is an important element in a number of Catholic groups. Some meet together at times, and the meeting closes with the singing of Compline. The singing may be not only devotional but also a beautiful rendition of the plain chant.

One should beware lest an emotional antagonism to "monasticism" should lead one to limit the freedom granted by the Church to individuals to choose at will approved private devotions to which they have a special attraction. To try to banish all group prayer from family life because it is "monastic" and incompatible with the Christian home would be to run counter to the officially expressed mind of the Church.

"The fathers and mothers of families particularly must give an example to their children, especially when, at sunset, they gather after the day's work, within the domestic walls, and recite the Holy Rosary on bended knees before the image of the Virgin, together fusing voice, faith and sentiment. This is a beautiful and salutary custom, from which certainly there cannot but be derived tranquility and abundance of heavenly gifts for the household."[9]

---

[7] Tertullian, *Apologia* Migne, P.L. I, 477.

[8] *The Epistles of St. Clement of Rome and St. Ignatius of Antioch.* Trans. by James A. Kleist, S. J. Newman, Westminster, Md. 1946, No. 12, p. 78.

[9] Pius XI, Encyclical Letter, Sept. 29, 1937: *On the Recitation of the Rosary to Combat Modern Evils.* National Catholic Welfare Conference, 1937, p. 10.

Now as to "extraordinary asceticism" we may say that heroic sanctity does not demand that either monks or members of the laity should have practiced extraordinary asceticism in order that their sanctity may be declared heroic and their beatification declared possible.[10]

Self-denial is looked upon as a virtue that belongs to those that go under the heading of Temperance. This means that its upper and lower limits must be determined in each individual with wise discretion. But as Benedict XIV points out, while the observance of nothing more than those things commanded by the Church (such as abstinence from meat on Friday) suffices for eternal salvation, an earnest, reasonable practice of self-denial is necessary to reach the summit of Christian perfection.

Self-denial in little things—restraining idle curiosity, holding back a sharp answer, letting others have their way for the sake of peace— will count more in estimating heroic self-denial than severe bodily penances which might perhaps be associated with vanity. If it were clear that penances were practiced mainly to satisfy vanity, it would put an end to the proceedings for canonization.

4. The Cloister of the Home

The cloister of the home is a moral cloister and has no physical limits. It is maintained by the mutual love of the father, the mother and the children, a love of each member of the family for all the others. As a result, they desire to live together in the evenings whenever possible; to want to get back home when called away on business; to be all together, if it can be arranged, when away from home for the summer. Naturally this desire of each for all must, from time to time, be sacrificed, and, that too, more and more as the children grow older.

The cloister of the home was particularly strong in the family of St. Thomas More. Henry VIII enjoyed the brilliant humor of Sir Thomas so much that he was ever taking him away from his happy life with his children around the family fire. St. Thomas enjoyed his family more than the company of the king and contrived to get back to it. He "rendered his conversation as dull as he could devise it, grew slow in his answers and lagging with retorts. The ruse worked and the royal invitations ceased to shower. Then he went home joyfully and

---

[10] See Chapter XI: Human Reason and the Pleasures of Life.

sparkled at his own table in such wise as would have made the king open his heavy eyes to hear it."[11]

When a monk must leave the confines of his physical cloister, he goes first to receive his Abbot's blessing. In this way the physical cloister is extended and stretches spiritually and surrounds the monk with the protection of the Abbot's prayer, so long as he goes only where he received permission to go.

In our days a serious problem arises for parents in letting children go out at night, particularly adolescent girls. The parents should know the boy with whom a girl goes out, and she should go only to the place to which she has permission to go. And if she goes out with a group she must not swap partners. Obedience in this matter is only possible when from childhood on, a father or mother has developed a strong bond of affection with the child, made stronger still by spiritual ideals.

The cloister of the home is not a physical cloister. In the same sense, any of those unfortunates who have no home should cloister themselves in the wide open world by the Ten Commandments and the sound principles of a spiritual life.

Is the world outside the family godless and an enemy to the welfare of the family? The fact is that the world outside is made up of a mixture of good and wicked. Of the wicked world about us we can say what St. John said of the wicked, pagan world of his day. "Love not the world, nor the things that are in the world. If any man love the world, the charity of the Father is not in him. For all that is in the world is the concupiscence of the flesh and the consupiscence of the eyes and the pride of life, which is not of the Father, but is of the world." (I John II:15-16). It is from this world that parents must try to shield their adolescent children by rearing them to the love of the Eternal Father and loving obedience to their own parents, that the cloister of the home may be extended to protect them when the time comes when they must take their place as God's Knights in the warfare of the good with evil. All this does not prevent a family from taking part wisely in all civil duties.

The cloister of the home, like the monastery, is a *school of the service of God* in which the children are trained in every virtue. As we shall see in

---

11 Richard Lawrence Smith, *John Fisher and Thomas More*, London, Sheed and Ward, 1935, p. 91.

the chapters that follow, the acquisition of stable virtues is a powerful prophylactic against various mental disorders. A virtuous man has a strong, vigorous personality. Such a personality can bear up against the stress and strain of life and often remains at his duty when a weaker would have a mental breakdown.

In a monastery there is one, or perhaps two years novitiate, in which the young monk is trained in virtue. Nor does that training ever entirely cease. Usually the postulant has had a good deal of training in virtue before he applies. In fact, training in virtue is pre-eminently the function of the home; and one whose judgment is not warped by a monasterio-phobia will have no difficulty in seeing that the home, like the monastery, must be a school of the service of God in which souls are led on to heroic sanctity.

St. Benedict, the founder of Western Monasticism (480?-543), wrote thus: "We have, therefore, to establish a school of the Lord's service, in the setting forth of which we hope to order nothing that is harsh or rigourous. But if anything be somewhat strictly laid down, according to the dictates of sound reason, for the amendment of vices or the preservation of charity, do not therefore fly in dismay from the way of salvation, whose beginning cannot but be strait and difficult. But as we go forward in our life and in faith, we shall with hearts enlarged and unspeakable sweetness of love, run in the way of God's commandments so that never departing from His guidance, but persevering in the monastery until death, we may by patience share in the sufferings of Christ, that we may deserve to be partakers of His Kingdom. Amen."[12]

From these words of St. Benedict we can see that "extraordinary asceticism" need not form an element in monastic life. Nor is it implied when we say that a home, like a monastery, must be a school of the service of God.

How are children taught to observe *all the virtues*? *Not* by definition and didactic teaching. The parents must themselves be virtuous or the teaching will fail. In the early life of the child they teach by example, especially by the love, kindness, and patience which they show to each other and to the children. The impatient parent often gives the child

[12] Closing words of the Prologue to The Rule of St. Benedict, trans. by Dom Oswald Hunter Blair, Fort Augustus, Scotland, 1934. Printed and Published by the Abbey Press.

its first training in lying. A mother hears a crash, runs to the kitchen and sees one of her beautifully decorated platters on the floor all smashed to smithereens. She cries out in an angry manner to her frightened little one: "Did you do that?" What can the poor child say but, "No!" in spite of the fact that it is quite evident he did. But had the mother come in perfectly undisturbed and said to the child: "My dear child, you had a little accident, didn't you? Come and tell me about it." The child would have received its first lesson in telling the truth.

Parents should use all the great and little troubles of family life to perfect themselves and train the children in all the virtues. Love, patience, kindly explanations, encouragement will make any home what it should be, a school of the service of God.

The Abbot of a monastery and the brother cellarer, the father and the mother in the home, have certain traits in common. I have heard it often said that St. Benedict drew the ideal of an abbot from that of a good father in his home. (The word abbot means "father.") If that is so, one can pick out things in the rule of St. Benedict that will be guiding principles to a father.

With a happily married couple there is never any difficulty about who is going to be boss. St. Paul puts the whole matter of family relationships in a clear light:

"Wives be subject to your husbands, as it behooveth in the Lord.

Husbands love your wives and be not bitter towards them.

Children obey your parents in all things for this is well pleasing to the Lord.

Fathers provoke not your children to indignation, lest they be discouraged.

Servants obey in all things your masters according to the flesh; not serving to the eye as pleasing men, but in simplicity of heart, fearing God." (Col. III:18-22).

Where there is love there is no difficulty. The mother wants the father to use his authority as the head of a social unit of society to direct all things wisely. One takes pleasure in obeying one whom one loves above all others in the world. The father wants to make his wife the happiest woman in the world and would never grieve her under any circumstances.

Let us now paraphrase some passages in the rule of St. Benedict concerning the abbot:

The father should remember that he holds the place of Christ in the monastery. Therefore he ought not (God forbid) to teach or ordain or command anything contrary to the law of God.

He ought to govern his children by a two-fold teaching: that is, he should shew forth all goodness and holiness by his deeds rather than his words when his children are young, and later on, the way of right living should be also infused into the minds of his children by his *teaching,* like the leaven of divine justice.

Let him not shut his eyes to the faults of his children; but as soon as they appear let him strive with all his might to root them out, remembering the fate of Heli the priest of Silo.

Let him be certainly assured that on the Day of Judgment he will have to give an account to the Lord of the souls of all his children as well as his own. And thus being ever fearful of the coming inquiry which the Shepherd will make of the family committed to his care, while he is careful of the account his children will have to render, he will be solicitous also of his own. And so while correcting the children by his admonitions, he himself will be cured of his own defects.

But even in his corrections let him act with prudence and not go too far, lest while he seeketh too eagerly to scrape off the rust, the vessel be broken. Let him keep his own frailty ever before his eyes and remember that the bruised reed must not be broken.

Let him so temper all things that the strong may have something to strive for, and the weak nothing at which to take alarm. And especially let him observe in all things the words of Christ, so that having fulfilled his stewardship he may hear from the Lord what that good servant heard, who gave wheat to his fellow servants in due season: "Amen I say unto you, over all his goods shall he place him."[13]

There are many things in St. Benedict's instructions to the Abbot that apply also to the mother of a family. To a very large extent the instruction of the children devolves upon her, but the father should not rid himself entirely of the duty of training his children. Ordinarily the mother is also almost entirely responsible for management and regulation of household affairs. So what St. Benedict says of the duties of the brother cellarer have special meaning for the mother in her home.

"Let her have the care of everything but let all be known and approved by the father of the household.

---

[13] From Chapters II and LXIV in the Rule of St. Benedict, op. cit.

"If a child ask her for anything unreasonably let her not treat him with contempt and so grieve him, but reasonably and with all humility refuse what he asks for amiss. Let her be watchful over her own soul, remembering always that saying of the Apostle that he that hath ministered well purchaseth to himself a good degree. (I Tim. III:13).

"Let her above all things have humility; and to a child on whom she hath nothing to bestown, let her give at least a kind answer, as it is written: a good word is above the best gift. (Eccl. XVIII:17). Let the meals be served on time without delay and making a fuss.

"Let her arrange all things that no one may be troubled or grieved in the home which should be in peace and quiet like the house of God."[14]

The ideal home is one in which the parents are striving for that heroic sanctity which God asks of all, and in so doing they lead their children to the same high ideal. When circumstances allow, every morning sees the whole family at Mass and Holy Communion. Peace reigns in the household.

The prudence of the parents looks ahead. In various ways the children are led to conceive the ideal of equipping themselves to something worthwhile before God and man when they enter life, and not waste their years in the bewitching of trifling.

In this way, the cloister of the home brings about a permanent isolation of the soul from all that is not God. In God all His attributes are identical with His Essence. It is more true to say with St. John that God is Love, rather than that God loves. So in seeking to do only what God wills, and give up all He wills not, the soul becomes isolated from all that is not God; and still moves about doing good to men. All this is reasonable, for it means no more than to labor at all that concerns you: what God wills; and to give up all that concerns you not: what God does not will.

In this way one learns to fulfill perfectly, everywhere and at all times, all one's obligations to God and man. This is *Heroic Sanctity*. Let us now study it in detail.

---

[14] Paraphrased from The Rule of St. Benedict. Ch. XXXI, op. cit., pp. 95-97.

CHAPTER II

What is Sanctity?

THE PRESENT CHAPTER attempts to give a definite detailed answer to this question. The very concept of sanctity seems unknown to the psychiatrists of our day. Though more or less inadequate attempts have been made to study what is vaguely termed "religion" in relation to mental disorder, I know of no study of the relation of a high degree of sanctity to mental disorder.[1]

On the other hand many works on the spiritual life discuss sanctity under the name of perfection; and the larger treatises[2] give a detailed account of the Moral and Theological Virtues that one must acquire or have infused into him by God if he is going to attain to sanctity.

Every human being should realize that he is called by God to be perfect even as He is perfect: "Be you therefore perfect, as also your Heavenly Father is perfect." (Matthew V: 48). Every man therefore should do all in his power to be a saint and live on earth a beautiful life of charity that characterizes the saints in heaven. It is very unlikely that everyone who attains to the sanctity of the saints will be

---

[1] As an example of a concept of religion which is presented "as the major challenge which the mental hospital offers to the student of religion," one may take the study of Anton T. Boisen: "The Genesis and Significance of Mystical Identification in cases of Mental Disorder." *Psychiatry*, 15: 287-296, 1952. The basis of his study was 78 male patients, most of them schizophrenics. "Such patients believe that God talks to them or that the devil is on their trail. Many of them identify themselves with Christ or God and feel that they are charged with some prophetic mission." Such studies have nothing to do with sanctity and religion. This will become evident to anyone who reads this chapter.

As an example of the statistical point of view: the percentage of Catholics, Protestants and Jews in a given group of insane patients, we may take: Charles B. Farr and Revel I. Howe: "The Influence of Religious Ideas on Etiology, Symptomatology and Prognosis of the Psychoses." *Am. J. Psychiatry*, 77: 846-865, 1932. The very term *religious ideas* suggests, as is the case, that the *putting in practice of religious ideas and ideals* in a holy life is not considered.

[2] Such as Adolphe Tanquery, *The Spiritual Life*, 2nd Ed. Westminster, Md., Newman Press, 1930.

canonized. For Holy Mother Church can only canonize a few to serve as examples for the faithful. And many a holy soul after the winter of this life on first entering heaven will feel like the ugly duckling after the dreary winter in the swamp, when they hear the angels cry: O come all ye angels and saints of God, and see the beautiful soul who has just entered heaven.

Bearing these things in mind it will be well for everyone to shape his or her life to the making of a saint. To help them to do that we have analyzed the concept of heroic virtue that Benedict XIV shows us must be demonstrated in anyone the Church beautifies or canonizes. Perhaps the picture may also be helpful to psychiatrists who would study religion and sanctity in relation to mental disorder.

1. The Degree of Sanctity Required for Canonization

What degree of sanctity is required for canonization? This matter has been the subject of more theoretical discussion along with judicial proceedings than any other problem, perhaps, that the human mind has discussed. This seems to be an extreme statement. But note that "theoretical discussion" is conjoined with "judicial proceedings" in the statement. For centuries the problem has been discussed theoretically by many great theologians. And again and again candidates for beatification and canonization have been presented to the ecclesiastical courts. All their writings, published and unpublished, whether books or letters, have been gathered and carefully studied. Every possible shred of evidence on the manner of their living has been examined. Then all the evidence for and against beatification or canonization is discussed in an elaborate judicial process. The end is to determine whether or not the candidate in his life became a hero of virtue and a shining example to all.

The word hero comes to us from paganism. In paganism the term was given to those who were outstanding for some great deed. It was not necessary that the hero should be outstanding in every virtue. But in a candidate for beatification or canonization there can be no vice. Some virtues must exist in an *heroic* degree and all in at least a high degree.

2. What Must Be Proved

Benedict XIV quotes Cardinal de Laurea on this point: According to the practice of the Apostolic See, all the virtues must be proved.

"This is evident from the fact and practice of the Church, which in the beatification and canonization of saints who are proposed for our imitation, is not content with the proof of any one virtue, but requires proof of all though it is not necessary that the servant of God should have at all times practised them, nor that all of them should have been in the heroic degree, for St. Jerome thinks that never happened. It is sufficient however to know that those are considered perfect by the Church who had all the virtues, and that these are worthy of beatification."[3]

Somewhat more clear are the words of Benedict XIV, himself: "We must not, however, understand . . . that in every case of beatification and canonization, it is necessary to prove the existence of both the theological and cardinal virtues in the heroic degree, by manifold heroic acts of the same kind, proceeding from each of the virtues aforesaid: but that in every such case, by manifold heroic acts must be proved the existence of the theological virtues, and above all, of Charity, in the heroic degree."[4]

"The theological virtues having been proved in the manner aforesaid, it is necessary that the existence of the cardinal or moral virtues[5] should be proved, not always however, but sometimes by heroic actions and sometimes by ordinary ones, the necessity of the heroic actions being restricted to those virtues in which the servant of God, whilst he lived, was able to exercise himself according to his state and condition of life."[6] Some persons cannot exercise some of the moral virtues in a heroic degree. Thus a married woman cannot practise virginity which is a part of the virtue of chastity which belongs to the moral virtue of temperance.[7]

3. Special Characteristics of Heroic Virtue

We may now attempt to outline the special characteristics of heroic acts of virtue.

It is not sufficient to demonstrate a single or a number of acts of

---

[3] *Heroic Virtue. A Portion of the Treatise of Benedict XIV on the Beatification and Canonization of the Servants of God.* Trans. by the Fathers of the Congregation of the Oratory. London. Thomas Richardson 1850, I., p. 41. This great work was written before Prospero Lambertini became Benedict XIV.

[4] Benedict XIV, *Heroic Virtue.* op. cit. I, p. 28.

[5] Prudence, justice, temperance, fortitude, and their associated virtues.

[6] *Heroic Virtue,* I, p. 30.

[7] St. Thomas *Summa Theologica* 2.2. Q. CLI and CLII.

outstanding merit such as, for instance, to give a vast fortune in charity and enter a religious order—but with great effort of will and also with regrets. It must be evident that heroic acts arise from a well-established habit. "Excellence in virtues cannot be said to be proved by acts, unless such acts were elicited easily and with delight."[8]

Heroic virtue "never allows of anything low, anything mean, or any even pardonable imperfection of manners, on full deliberation, but at all times and places retains that sublimity of soul, tending with all its might to the highest goodness, and to the following of God."[9] There are, however, degrees in the might of God's heroes.

The degrees of "might" in God's heroes raises the question of the extent to which "absolute virtue" is realized in human beings. Every virtue is an ideal, even as every person is an ideal that exists in the eternal immutable Essence of the Divine Nature. This ideal of a virtue may be termed "absolute virtue" or the exemplar of virtue in the mind of God. Such virtue can only be approached but never attained by any creature.

The highest attainable virtue for man is sometimes termed the virtue of a "purified soul." Years have passed since the soul commenced seriously to strive for spiritual perfection. In all this time the hero has remained ever the same in the sense that he never strayed from the path of virtue.[10] Many and severe have been the trials of life. And as the years rolled on there was not only no complaint but also in every trial perfect patience, peace, joy and humility. Finally, the peace became continuous both in joy and in sorrow. And in the peace a light shone through a veil and the soul knew the presence of its Creator. Though that light waxed and waned, it was never extinguished. And with the light there developed perfect emotional control. The soul had been purified. God's grace flowed into intellect and will and no unworthy emotion could disturb the peace of the soul. All such emotions were promptly banished as soon as they appeared. The soul lived in perfect union with Christ, its Eternal Spouse.

Benedict XIV, quoting St. Thomas, says: "The virtues of a soul already purified exist in such wise that prudence gazes only on things

---

[8] *Heroic Virtue*, op. cit. I, p. 32.
[9] *Heroic Virtue*, op. cit. I, p. 33.
[10] Loc. cit.

divine, temperance knows no earthly longings, fortitude is ignorant of
passion, justice is allied to the Divine mind by a perpetual covenant."[11]

4. *The Sanctity of St. Paul, the Apostle*

Virtues that do not rise to the perfection of the virtues of a purified
soul but lead to them are termed *virtues of purification*. Is it true that
heroic virtue necessarily implies the virtues of a purified soul or is the
heroism of *long continued* and *successful* combat true heroism and is it
sufficient for canonization?

We can make this matter clearer from the consideration of two
states in the spiritual development of St. Paul the Apostle.

St. Paul tells us, when writing his second Epistle to the Corinthians,
that "above 14 years ago he had wonderful revelations" and then he
says: "Lest the greatness of the revelations should exalt me, there was
given me a sting of the flesh an angel of Satan to buffet me."[12] It
would seem that at this period, shortly after his conversion, his were
the "virtues of purification."

Over fourteen years, therefore, before he wrote the second Epistle to
the Corinthians, he had not yet attained to the virtues of a purified
soul. For in such a state the soul is risen to a sanctity that resembles
that of the Blessed Mother, in which it is no longer necessary to
struggle; for emotionality has been subjected to reason illumined by
divine grace.

But in his Epistle to the Galatians, written long after[13] the sting of
the flesh was imposed upon him, he writes: "With Christ, I am nailed
to the Cross, I live now, not I, but Christ liveth in me. And that I live
now in the flesh: I live in the faith of the Son of God, who loved me

---

[11]*Heroic Virtue*, op. cit. p. 50. See St. Thomas, 1.2. Q. LXI.v. This is one of a number
of passages in St. Thomas in which he writes from personal experience. Its evidence
is due to its autobiographic character.

[12]II. Cor. xii, 7. This "sting of the flesh" has been interpreted by some as meaning
a physical disease. Conjectures range from gout to epilepsy. But the natural
interpretation of the words "an angel of Satan" requires the meaning: a temptation
hard to resist.

[13]Gal. ii, 1. He writes of going up to Jerusalem 14 years after his former visit to see
St. Peter 1 in Jerusalem. This second visit was therefore about 17 years from his con-
version. The Epistle to the Galatians was written during St. Paul's 2nd or 3rd
Missionary Journey, that is between 50 and 58 A.D., more probably towards 58.
John E. Steinmueller: *A Companion to Scripture Studies*. New York. 1943, III, pp. 260-
261.

and delivered himself for me."[14] These words may well be taken to mean that at the time he wrote them the sting of the flesh was gone and all emotions and desires were subject to Christ who lived in him to such an extent that he no longer seemed to live independently of Christ to whom he was entirely subject without any shadow of rebellion.

We have, therefore, two states of the spiritual life: a first in which there is a severe but *entirely successful* conflict with passion. Satan attacks fiercely but he is just as fiercely attacked and routed. It is a state of combat, but without sin—*a state of being purified* by fidelity in time of trial.

The second is one in which the power of the soul has been so strengthened by Christ, in reward for long, fierce, and faithful combat to maintain spiritual ideals, that all unworthy emotions are promptly banished. They cannot tarry a moment in the mind of the now *purified soul.*

Does heroic virtue demand the *state of the purified soul?* Or will the *state of being purified suffice?* If heroic virtue demands the first, then St. Paul in spite of his heroism in sacrificing all that was dear to him to follow Christ, and his heroic preaching of Christ, and his heroic battle against the sting of the flesh, could not have been "canonized" had he died before he attained the state in which he no longer lived, but Christ lived in him. This state is regarded by theologians as that of the Blessed in Heaven.

Benedict XIV cites several good theologians who held that the virtues of a purified soul are necessary for canonization. But he himself thinks that very few saints have attained on earth to the perfection of the Blessed in Heaven, and regards the heroism of living in ever successful conflict with all manner of temptations as heroism sufficient for canonization.[15]

5. A Definition of Heroic Sanctity

Throughout all definitions of sanctity must run the example and teaching of Christ who did the will of His Father in heaven. The definition of sanctity must make clear the identity between the doing

---

[14]Gal. ii, 19-20. A. Robert and A. Tricot (*Guide to the Bible,* Eng. Trans., Tournai, Desclée, 1951) adopt the same view and say, "It was maintained in antiquity by St. Jerome." II, pp. 231-232.

[15]Op. cit. I, p. 59: "It is not necessary for heroic virtue to be that of the purified soul."

of the will of God and the keeping of His commandments: "If any man love Me, he will keep my commandments." (John XIV:23).

Sanctity must be open to all. It does not demand a heroism that only the rich and powerful can display. Of all heroism, that is the most sublime and difficult which passes through the temptations of life without ever having committed a mortal or even a fully deliberate venial sin.

Considerations such as these perhaps led Benedict XV to give the following definition of sanctity:[16] *Sanctity properly consists in simple conformity to the Divine Will expressed in an exact fulfillment of the duties of one's proper state.*

The definition of Benedict XV makes true sanctity open to all, but it does not make it any easier to attain. It will, however, stimulate many to take up its pursuit precisely because it is the greatest of all goods and within the grasp of anyone who asks the help of God, tries his best to get it, and never gives up.

6. Spiritual Marriage and the Virtues of a Purified Soul

It may well be said that the state of *spiritual marriage* and the possession of the *virtues of a purified soul* differ only in name.

(a) One who has attained to the virtues of a purified soul, says St. Thomas, sees everything from the point of view of God.[17] In spiritual matrimony with Christ the soul can live in an unbroken consciousness of the presence of the Blessed Trinity. Thus in 1581 in a "relation" of the state of her soul to her former confessor Don Alonso Velasquez (by that time Bishop of Osmo), St. Teresa of Avila writes: "The imaginary visions have ceased, but I seem always to be having this intellectual vision of the three Divine Persons and of Christ's Humanity, which I think is of a much higher kind."[18] In such a condition a soul could not but see all things from the point of view of God.

(b) In spiritual matrimony[19] and in the purified soul there is an

---

[16]Made in the allocution accompanying the promulgation in 1916 of the heroism of Jean Baptiste de Burgogne. Quoted from Père Gabriele de Ste. Marie-Madeleine. *Present Norms of Holiness in Conflict and Light,* edited by Père Bruno de Jesu-Marie, O.C.D., New York, Sheed and Ward, 1952, p. 158. Père Gabriele's study is based on his experience in the Congregation of Rites during processes of canonization.

[17]1.2, Q. LXI, v. corpus. St. Thomas here says of the justice of the purified soul: "Justice is united with the divine mind in a perpetual covenant" and then adds, "by imitating it." In St. Teresa of Avila the union was also conscious: an abiding intellectual vision of the three Divine Persons.

[18]Peer's translation. I, p. 335. Relation VI in 1581. St. Teresa died Oct. 4, 1582.

[19]St. John of the Cross. Spiritual Canticle. Stanzas XX and XXI (second redaction) Peers Translation, II, p. 296.

abiding unbroken peace. St. Thomas compares the state of the
purified soul to that of the Blessed in heaven or to that of a certain few
on this earth at the height of spiritual perfection.[20]

(c) In the state of spiritual matrimony the soul closely resembles
Christ in Whom no unworthy emotion could appear in the field of
consciousness. St. John expresses this by using "first movements" to
indicate the appearance of any mental activity in the field of consciousness. All the mental faculties "tend in their first movements,
without the soul's being conscious of it, to work in God and through
God. For the understanding the will and the memory go straightway
to God; and the affections, the senses, the desires and appetites, hope,
enjoyment and the rest of the soul's possessions are inclined to God
from the first movement even though, as I say, the soul may not
realize that it is working for God."[21] Hence the soul is no longer
troubled by distractions in prayer.

St. Thomas says: "that in the purified soul temperance knows no
cravings and fortitude experiences no emotions."[22]

It would seem that St. Teresa and St. John of the Cross in describing
the state of spiritual matrimony are giving merely a more complete
account and illustration of what St. Thomas calls the virtues of a
purified soul. St. John of the Cross says of spiritual matrimony: "I
think that this estate is never attained without the soul being confirmed in grace therein . . . Wherefore this is the loftiest estate which
in this life is attainable."[23]

As we have noted, (page 17), Benedict XIV holds that the state of a
purified soul is not demanded for canonization and few canonized
saints have ever attained it. Does God call all men to attain to the
virtues of a purified soul and spiritual matrimony, or only a certain
few and, therefore, not all, even of the canonized saints, are called to
the heights of perfection?

Our Lord's own words tell us that He calls all men to the highest
possible sanctity that can be attained. His Sermon on the Mount was
spoken to the common people and therefore meant for all. And He
said therefore to every Christian: "Be you therefore perfect as also your
heavenly Father is perfect." (Matthew V:48). There is no such thing
as two classes of Christians, an upper and a lower. All are called to the

---

[20]Loc. cit. [21]*Spiritual Canticle* XXVIII, Peer's trans. II, p. 343.
[22]Loc. cit. [23]*Spiritual Canticle* XXII (2nd redaction) Peer's trans. II, p. 308.

same heights of perfection and these heights are attainable in any state or condition of life.

To solve this difficulty we must consider what the mystic graces, of which spiritual matrimony is the greatest, do for us: They help us to attain our end more easily.[24] Charity is the attainment of our end:[25] the union with God in love. One who makes full use of his mystic graces will advance more quickly in the way of divine charity. But by the mere fact that one has received mystic graces he is not more holy than one who has not received them. The peace and freedom from emotional disturbance of spiritual matrimony is a reward for past merit gained in the fierce struggle to attain the *purifying* virtues. Some saints, for reasons known to God alone, commence to receive their eternal reward, in part, even in this life and attain to the peace of spiritual matrimony. Others must wait until they see God face to face in eternal glory and "shall be like to Him *because* they shall see Him as He is." (I John III:2). But as Benedict XIV shows, there are degrees of perfection in heroic sanctity; and some will attain to spiritual matrimony because of a more purifying struggle in the attainment of heroic virtue. But it may be possible that some great heroes among the canonized saints must, because God so wills it, wait for their spiritual matrimony with Christ for the final purification of the beatific vision.

Should every soul throughout life hold constantly in mind the attainment of the virtues of a purified soul? We *must*, if we are going to obey the injunction of Christ *to be perfect even as our heavenly Father is perfect.* We must, therefore, in all our contacts with others throughout life have before our minds the society of the Blessed in heaven. Remember that if a saint from heaven could come to earth and play your part in life for a while he would manage with perfect peace of mind all those acute incidents in which you display so many and such undesirable emotions.

If you look at a photograph of a battleship steaming into action, you will see the big guns pointed upward as if to shoot at the moon. Aim at the virtues of the Blessed in heaven and you will attain to the heroism of the saints on earth.

---

[24]They are what St. Thomas calls *gratiae gratis datae* which put a man in touch with something preparatory to his final end.

[25]It is what St. Thomas calls a *gratia gratum faciens*; it relates man immediately to his end. 1.2, Q. CXI, v, corpus.

CHAPTER III

Heroic Faith

1. The Theological Notion of Faith

Benedict XIV in his discussion of Faith takes St. Paul's definition as his starting point: "Faith is the substance of things to be hoped for and the evidence of things that appear not." (Hebrews XI:1). It is the exact expression, the very substance of all we hope for in eternal life. Its object is God the First Truth on Whom all other truths depend. It brings us face to face with God and our relations to Him not merely in time but also in eternity. In the act of faith God illumines the mind to understand what is meant by the substance of all we hope for and at the same time inclines the will to accept what we believe, not by scientific or logical reasoning, but because God the First Truth has revealed it. This illumination of the mind and inspiration of the will is the evidence of the things that appear not.[1]

"Abraham believed God and it was reputed to him unto justice." (Genesis XV:6). Faith, therefore, is a meritorious act leading to true sanctity and eternal life. It must, therefore, be a free and responsible act. "Our acts are meritorious in so far as they proceed from free will moved by God through grace."[2]

In all voluntary acts the good that is sought, chosen, and loved organizes the mind and all its activities in seeking it. But in faith it is God Who is sought and to live with Him in the perfect union of love in eternal life. This organization of the mind, in the act of faith by the love of God, is spoken of by theologians as *fides formata:* formed or organized faith. Should the soul fall into grievous sin, the habit of faith would no longer be organized by divine charity. It would not be destroyed but it would become *fides informis:* unformed or unorganized faith.

---

[1] St. Thomas, *Summa Theologica.* 2.2. Q. IV, i, Corpus. St. Thomas here reformulates the definition of St. Paul thus: Faith is a habit of the mind by which eternal life is commenced within us making the intellect assent to things that appear not.

[2] St. Thomas. 2.2. Q. II, ix, Corpus.

2. Canonical Process of Determining Heroic Faith

How does the Church go about determining whether or not a candidate for canonization has faith in a high or even in a heroic degree?

The procedure is based on the discussion of faith and works by St. James in his Epistle: "Even as the body without the spirit is dead, so also faith without works is dead." (James II:26).

Living faith is the cause of the good works in a man's life. And as the load an engine can pull measures the power of an engine, so the good works a man performs measure the vigor of his faith.

The Church does not attempt to read the thoughts of men nor to measure directly the vigor of their living faith. It turns to *deeds done* that unmistakably bear witness to the power of the living faith within. Thus, when Our Lord was dying on the Cross, one of the two thieves beside Him took up the mockery of the rabble around them. The other rebuked him and then turned to Jesus and said: "Lord, remember me when Thou shalt come into Thy Kingdom." (St. Luke XXIII:42). In all the history of Christianity there was no more heroic act of faith. There could be no doubt of a faith that had already sanctified Our Lord's companion in death and had risen in a moment to the utmost heights of faith and of humility.

What are the deeds that manifest faith? Faith involves both intellect and will. There will be, therefore, two types of activities that will demonstrate faith. Thus the writings of the great theologians such as the *Summa* of St. Thomas Aquinas are lasting testimonials to the greatness of their faith. And the fearless penetration of St. Francis Xavier alone and without escort into the heart of sixteenth century Japan was a witness to his heroic faith.

The Revelations of Divine Love showed to Mother Juliana of Norwich bear witness to the intellectual side of her faith. She speaks of the knowledge she had of the faith from the common teaching of the Church. And a knowledge that was given to her of the Church's doctrines that was "endless continuant love with sureness of keeping and blissful salvation." There was no difference whatsoever between the teaching in her revelations (showings) and that of the common teaching of the Church which she had learned in childhood.[3] In other

---

[3] *Revelations of Divine Love Showed to Mother Juliana of Norwich.* 1373. Preface by George Tyrrell, S.J. London. Kegan Paul, etc., 1920, p. 11.

words, the revelations gave her a vastly deeper penetration into some of the teachings of the Church and so her Faith became richer.

3. Ways in Which God Illumines the Mind

We might here remark that Faith is always begotten by God illuminating the intellect but there are various ways in which this is done. Generally, perhaps, this illumination does not seem to come directly from God. One hears a sermon that for some reason has a powerful effect on the soul, or one reads a book and starts to think seriously on God and our duties to our Creator. But then there are illuminations that seem to come more and more clearly directly from God, pointing to the Church as His divine institution or directing souls to lead a saintly life. Then again, the soul suddenly feels that God is talking to it, whether by a flow of ideas or by spoken words may not be clear; but what is said brings about of itself a real change for the better.[4] Let us illustrate from the spiritual history of St. Thérèse of Lisieux.

"About this time (shortly after her miraculous cure [see page 216]) I received what I have looked on as one of the greatest graces of my life, for at that age, I was not favored with lights from heaven, as I am now.

Our Lord made me understand that the only true glory is that which lasts forever; and that to attain it there is no necessity to do brilliant deeds, but rather to hide oneself from the eyes of others, and even from oneself, so that the left hand knows not what the right hand does."[5]

Further on in her biography she refers to these lights from heaven that she mentions in the above quotation. After saying that the works of spiritual writers no longer interested her and that she found in the Holy Scriptures and the *Imitation* her greatest help, she continues:

---

[4] What St. John of the Cross would term "substantial words." *Ascent of Mount Carmel.* Book II, Chapter XXXI.

[5] The first paragraph in the quotation is as found in the manuscript. The second and the two following paragraphs have been modified; but the(essential meaning is not altered. See *Manuscript* p. 32, right. (Manuscript refers here and elsewhere to the facsimile reproduction *Manuscrits Autobiographiques,* Carmel de Lisieux, 1956. The right-hand page only is numbered; hence, right refers to the numbered page; and left, to the unnumbered. The usual designation is R⁰—right; V⁰—left (unnumbered).) The passage quoted is from T. N. Taylor's translation *Soeur Thérèse of Lisieux.* New York, Kenedy, 1924, p. 55.

"Our Lord has no need of books or teachers to instruct our souls. He, the Teacher of Teachers, instructs us without any noise of words. . I have never heard Him speak, yet I know He is within me. He is there, always guiding and inspiring me; and just when I need them, lights hitherto unseen, break in. This is not as a rule during my prayers, but in the midst of my daily duties."[6]

It is a fundamental teaching of St. John of the Cross that Faith not only teaches about God but by Faith the soul journeys to God.[7] But the difficulty in general is that few saints leave autobiographies sufficiently complete to let us know to what extent they received and followed the guidance of God in all they did. But St. Thérèse of Lisieux has given us sufficient insight into her following of God by Faith to show that her faith was heroic. Benedict XIV says of heroic virtue that "it never allows of anything low, anything mean, or any even pardonable imperfection of manners, on full deliberation, but at all times and places retains that sublimity of soul, tending with all its might to the highest goodness, and to the following of God."[8] This was true of Saint Thérèse from childhood in ever-increasing fullness on to her death.

But the Church would never canonize any one on the basis of an autobiography. Sanctity must be demonstrated by good deeds of *all* the virtues possible for the candidate to practice. Once, however, sanctity has been demonstrated independently by deeds, all the writings of the one to be canonized are carefully scrutinized. On the principle that one who practices all the virtues would not give a lying account of himself, light may be thrown on his inner spiritual life by an autobiography.

Benedict XIV gives in detail what special points are raised in demonstrating the existence of the ordinary habit of theological Faith.

1. Did the candidate openly confess those things which are believed in the heart by faith: especially when circumstances demanded an open confession?

2. Did the candidate keep the Commandments?

3. Did the candidate pray to God?

4. Did the candidate manifest submission of the heart and obedience

---

[6] Taylor's translation, p. 131. Manuscript 84, left. Translation, after the word "inspiring" omits "ce que je dois dire ou faire."

[7] *Spiritual Canticle.* Stanza I, 11. Peer's translation Vol. II, p. 199.

[8] *Heroic Virtue*, op. cit. I, p. 33.

to God, to the Catholic Church, and its visible head, the Roman Pontiff, in all things which must be believed and done for eternal salvation?

5. Did the candidate's faith increase or did he at least desire its increase?

6. Did he have the fear of God?

7. Did he adore God and honor His saints?

8. Did he have a horror for sin and do penance if he fell into sin?[9]

9. Did he show patience in the trials of life?

10. Did he have joy in carrying out good works, in humility and in humiliations?[10]

Heroic faith is "discerned by the same acts, that is, if there be a frequency in their performance, if they are accompanied with ease, readiness, and pleasurable feeling,[11] and if in the circumstances under which they are done there be something eminently arduous, to excite admiration, and so to elevate the agent above the ordinary manner of working, even of good men."[12]

4. Examples of Heroic Faith

Benedict XIV quotes as examples: The certainty of the Faith of *St. Teresa of Avila* which no other certainty could approach. Her knowledge of the Divine Presence was so clear that it was akin to vision. *St. Peter of Alcantara* had a similar certainty of faith. *St. Paschal Baylon*, though uneducated, wrote on the basis of his faith, about heavenly things, particularly the mystery of our redemption. Thus, God had lifted him to the heights of the intellectual element in faith, even though he was uneducated.

The following account of the spiritual life of a day laborer, because of its richness in little details, will give a vivid picture of what may ultimately be heroic faith.

---

[9] There are two ways to canonization: (1) The way of innocence which those trod who never stained their baptismal robe by a single mortal sin all throughout life. (2) The way of penance which was entered sometime after their fall. But there must have been a period before death during which they never slipped into even a venial sin after due reflection.

[10] Somewhat abbreviated from Benedict XIV, *Heroic Virtue* I, pp. 81-82.

[11] It seems to the author that "delight" as used elsewhere in the book would be a better translation, though he has not seen the original. "Feeling" might indicate a sensory reaction. But the reaction is to what intellect alone can perceive, not to what any of the senses can be aware of.

[12] Op. cit., p. 82.

A day laborer happened to be given a job which was near a small old downtown Catholic church. At the time he was in a stage of the spiritual life which Abbot Chautard terms *moderate piety*. In this stage one slips easily into mortal sin, but is genuinely sorry and makes a good confession. Venial sin does not bother those in this stage. In general they know nothing about mental prayer, but occasionally say devoutly some vocal prayers.

It occurred to the day laborer that it might be a good thing to get up a little earlier and go to Mass every morning at the little downtown church. This was one of those illuminating graces that not only put an idea into the head but is also accompanied by an inspiring grace to carry it out in practice. We have seen (above, page 24) that one of the signs of true faith is to keep the commandments. To follow promptly good advice that comes from within is an even stronger sign. Soon came another piece of good interior advice. Go to Communion every morning. It was at once carried out.

The next grace was what theologians term an external grace. (See below, page 180.) At the rear of the Church he noticed a well-stocked pamphlet rack. The pamphlets "were a convenient and ever-ready source of information concerning Jesus, Our Lady, the saints and all manner of problems in religion and the spiritual life." A hard-working day laborer cannot well take a series of courses in dogmatic and ascetical theology for the laity; but he can read pamphlets.

He thus expresses the way in which God developed the virtue of faith in his soul: "With attendance at daily Mass and with daily communion and spiritual communion, my heart and mind have turned from worldly things to those of spirit and truth."

"In this way he passed from Chautard's third to his sixth stage[13] of the spiritual life and seems to be solidly established in an interior life of the soul with God. He makes no mention of any persons having played a role in the change that came over him." His daily life is now well-leavened. "My mental prayer," he writes, "has not followed any systematic plan. It has been chiefly a monologue in which I have thanked God for His favors and blessings and asked Him for further favors. Sometimes at prayer his whole being is infused with the love of God, and the peace of prayer follows him into the work of the day."

His self-denial, considering that his work is entirely rather heavy manual labor, might be termed vigorous. "No eating between meals,

---

[13]See T. V. Moore, *The Life of Man With God*, New York, Harcourt Brace, 1956, p. 387.

usually no breakfast, no movies nor radio programs. Rather seldom look at T.V. Place fifty cents in a mite box daily and when the coins have accumulated give them to the Society for the Propagation of the Faith. Rise at 4.30 a.m. Sundays, to serve Masses in a distant parish church." His life is not without mystic graces, such as, "It seems as if Christ were standing on my right side, as I knelt in prayer and He was placing His left Hand over my head."

His life has now been free for some time not only from mortal sin but also from all deliberate venial sin.

But we cannot say as yet that this day laborer has heroic faith. If, however, he perseveres on his present level, without slipping back and especially if he rises to even higher levels, and tends with all his might to the highest goodness and the following of God to the very end, he will die in the possession of heroic faith.

CHAPTER IV

The Theological Virtue of Hope

1. The Concept of Hope

"Hope is a supernatural infused virtue, by which, with reliance on God's Omnipotence, Goodness, and Fidelity, we look forward to eternal salvation and the necessary means to obtain it."[1]

Hope is termed a supernatural virtue because it cannot, like the natural moral virtues, be attained in any way by the unaided efforts of intellect and will. It is a theological virtue because it has God for its immediate object. It is an infused virtue because it is not acquired but infused with the bestowal of sanctifying grace at baptism. The salvation we look forward to is our union with God in heaven and the vision of Him face to face throughout all eternity.

We can "look forward" only to that about which we have some knowledge. The existence of hope depends, therefore, upon the knowledge of God given to us by *Faith*.

That to which we "look forward" we desire. There are two types of desire in the human mind: one of things perceived by the senses; the other of things that intellect alone can know. The craving for sensory things is sensory desire; that for intellectual things is an act of the will and not a sensory desire.[2]

Hope, therefore, is an abiding habit of the will by which one tends to seek and look forward to union with God for all eternity.

To enter heaven we must try to live a good life and avoid all sin. This is not an easy task. Furthermore, even if after a long life without serious effort to avoid sin we should repent and be saved on our death-bed, the purification of purgatory would await us before entrance into eternal life. Hope, therefore, looks forward to something difficult to attain in the future.

Like the laborers in the Gospel, man looks forward to the passing of

---

[1] Heribert Jone, O.F.M. Cap. *Moral Theology.* English Translation, Westminster, Md., Newman, 1955, § 129, p. 72-73.

[2] St. Thomas *Summa Theologica*, 2.2. Q. XVIII, i.

the heat and the burden of the day, and beyond the day of our life on earth he hopes for his reward in eternal life.

2. *Those Who Do Not Hope and Those Who Do*

Let us cast a glance now at the world as it actually is:

We find in the world throughout all history a large number of men who have no hope for any reward after the burden of the day and its heat are over. Their reward comes to them with their pay check. When that ceases at death, there is nothing more. Such a one once told me that his idea of a happy death would consist in enjoying a gorgeous ride in an airplane, going faster than sound, and having it unexpectedly crash into the Rock of Gibraltar.

But there are others who have the rudiments of Christian hope, but are still held captive by the fleshpots of Egypt. I was talking to one of these many years ago: "You know," he said, "I am perfectly satisfied with my life as it is. I would have no desire to go to heaven, if I could live on day after day, enjoying what I now enjoy, if I knew I would never grow any older and would never die." He was a fairly wealthy Catholic and yet was content with this concept of natural beatitude, such as many theologians postulate for children who die without baptism.

There was, however, in this wealthy man a hidden faith and a *latent* hope, for he went to Mass every Sunday and led a good moral life. There are many well-to-do Catholics whose faith and hope do not develop further than that of this wealthy man. They do not see further into their religion and have not experienced anything of the depths of the inner life of the soul with God. They love social functions, the theatre, traveling, good living and nice homes. None of these things are in themselves morally wrong. But to know God and live with Him and look forward constantly to our life with Him in eternity, while we carry out a mission for Him on earth, is something infinitely beyond the natural beatitude of the morally good who keep the Ten Commandments. Most of these good rich people would be hurt and surprised if any one accused them of not being good Catholics. For they keep the Ten Commandments and the precepts of the Church. It is true also that they seldom or never slip into mortal sin. But in all probability they do have a latent implicit hope. For they probably do not expect to avoid sin by their own native strength of will, but with the aid of grace which God will surely give if they ask for it. But they thoroughly enjoy the good pleasures of life and think seldom of the beatific vision in heaven.

What is lacking in the class of people we have just considered is a Eucharistic life of daily Mass and Holy Communion along with what St. Teresa of Avila terms that intimate friendship with God that comes with mental prayer. They have the opportunity and the time for a beautiful interior life but do not make use of it. This does not by any means signify that the interior life is absent in all who enjoy wealthy leisure. God has his saints in every walk and station of life.

The development of the interior life involves the growth of the theological virtues of faith, hope, and charity. In this inner life of the soul with God, the Holy Spirit causes His illuminating grace to shine upon the mind. Faith thus commences to teach the soul more and more about God and His love for man. Then hope transcends the condition of its latency and the soul explicitly, and with full consciousness, yearns to be united with God in heaven and behold Him face to face throughout all eternity. Then divine charity commences to glow; for already the mind sees in part, through a glass and in a dark manner, and the soul loves that which it has commenced to see. Both the Council of Trent and St. Thomas Aquinas teach us that faith absolutely precedes hope; and in order of birth hope is prior to charity.[3]

Latent hope leads one to do his best to avoid mortal sin and so get to heaven even while one enjoys intensely the innocent pleasures of the world. It may be looked upon as the lowest degree of the virtue of hope. One passes to a higher degree as we have said by commencing to lead a devout interior spiritual life. When we think of developing the virtue of hope we must remember that it is a theological virtue. That means that it is bestowed originally by God and that it can be increased only by God Himself. But when we do all we can God rewards our puny efforts by strengthening our hope in Him and our desire to see Him face to face for all eternity.

3. How We May Increase Our Hope

How shall we go about doing all we can on our part? Remember the words of St. Benedict, "In the first place, whatever good work thou beginnest to do, beg of God with most earnest prayer to perfect."[4] It

---

[3] Benedict XIV *Heroic Virtue*, Eng. Trans. I, 92. St. Thomas 2.2. Q. XVII, VII and VIII; Conc. Trid. Sessio VI, Caput 6, D.B. 798.
[4] Prologue of the Rule.

might be well also to turn our minds in our spare moments to think about our life with God in heaven. It will not be long before I pass from time to eternity. In that moment I shall appear before Christ Whom I have loved and served all the days of my life or since my heart gave itself wholly to Him. And if I shall have finally learned to live without any fully deliberate venial sin, I may hope to hear from Him: "Well done thou good and faithful servant, because thou hast been faithful over a few things, I will place thee over many things. Enter thou into the joy of the Lord." (Matthew XXV:21).

And then Christ will take a veil away from my mind and I shall behold in clearest intellectual vision Him in Whose immediate presence I have ever lived. And I shall be like Him because I shall see Him as He is. (See I John III:2). If the mystic knowledge of the divine presence which is sometimes granted us on earth causes such transcendent happiness, what will be the overwhelming joy of the soul that sees God face to face? And still though the joy will be overwhelming it will not overwhelm and the soul will be able to take part in the heavenly liturgy and sing the praises of the Creator with the nine choirs of angels and all the saints of the ages.

Then remember that you must first leave the earthly to draw near to the heavenly. And this we do when we pass from the stage of praying at certain times and pass on to that in which we shall live with God in a life of prayer. This will enable us to give up everything that does not concern us.

Persevere and there will come a time in your spiritual life when it will be possible to say of you truly that with God's help you have freed yourself from all earthly desires and have no longer any interest except in God and what He wants you to do in your life. When this point is reached you will arrive at the level of *heroic* hope.

But there are degrees in the heroism of the virtues. A soul such as we have just described will already be a "little" hero of the virtue of hope. It can go much further. It may sometime arrive at a stage when it not only yearns to be with God in heaven, but also finds it painful to remain on earth because its craving to be with God in heaven is so intense.

A number of members of the laity attain to this height of heroic hope. One wrote me that since she was about 17 it has been painful for her to be separated from Christ in heaven. It would seem that such souls have arrived at what St. Paul spoke of when he wrote: "For me to live in Christ and to die is gain . . . I am straitened between two: having a desire to be dissolved and to be with Christ, a thing by far the better. But to abide still in the flesh is needful to you." (Phil. I:21-24). Thus we see also that a yearning to be with Christ in heaven may coexist with a desire to serve Him on earth.

In St. Teresa of Avila the pain of separation from Christ in heaven became so acute, at times, that she thought she was actually on the point of expiring. She wrote thus: "It sometimes happens that when a person is in this state . . . and has such yearnings to die, because the pain is more than she can bear, that her soul seems to be on the very point of leaving the body, she is really afraid and would like her distress to be alleviated, lest she should in fact die."[5]

It would seem thus that we have certain stages of hope from its complete absence on to the heights of its perfection. These are:

1. *Absence of hope,* because of no belief in immortality.
2. *Latent hope,* which begins with an earnest striving to avoid mortal sin.
3. *Explicit hope,* when the soul is practicing a devout spiritual life, and often during mental prayer, or at any time in the day, turns with yearning to the thought of eternity and its future union with Christ and enjoyment of the beatific vision.
4. *Heroic hope,* when the soul, by the grace of God has freed itself from all earthly desires and no longer has any interest in what does not pertain to God and His service. Hope fixes the will on the vision of God in eternity while Love, granted the veiled vision of divinity, already is united with its Beloved on earth.

There are various degrees in this stage, culminating with an intensity of yearning for Christ that seems, for a time, to bring the soul to the point of leaving the body.

4. Objective Signs of the Existence of Hope

Benedict XIV speaks thus concerning the objective criteria of hope: "Putting aside, therefore, internal acts of which (as we have said) the Church doth not judge, a habit of hope, in the causes of the servants of God, may be presumed from external acts."[6] He then mentions the following external acts or types of behavior which have been used in the Roman courts to show *heroic* hope.

The great labors that the servants of God have undertaken for His sake and the severity of their penitential life. Such labors and penances

[5] *Interior Castle, VI,* xi. Peer's Trans. II, p. 327.
[6] Op. cit., p. 92.

would never be undertaken without hope in eternal life: Entrance into a religious order with surrender of all temporal goods, especially when this involves great property and positions of high dignity. Joy at the news of approaching death. The patience of martyrs in their torments. Joy in adversity. The special confidence that some of the saints have had that God would suddenly come to their aid when no aid seemed possible and which was confirmed by the event.

We may illustrate this last sign from the life of St. Vincent de Paul. From 1628 to 1639 Lorraine had suffered a series of misfortunes that reduced the whole country to a state of starvation. It was said that the land suffered more even than the inhabitants of Jerusalem during the siege of the Romans before its utter destruction. A letter by a priest tells of seeing more than a hundred starving creatures "who look like skeletons covered with skin . . . Their skin is like black marble and is so shrunken that their teeth are dry and uncovered, and their eyes and whole countenance have a scowling appearance."

In 17th century France there was no royal organization corresponding to our modern Red Cross to send into Lorraine and organize relief. St. Vincent de Paul learned of the state of affairs and he and his missionary priests, with money that St. Vincent collected, organized a truly vast project for the relief of a whole country that was literally starving to death.

Someone pointed out the distress of the noblemen of Lorraine whose castles had been destroyed, and they were compelled to leave Lorraine and live in poverty in Paris. Nobles could not beg. St. Vincent organized a group of wealthy noblemen, who promised to get a monthly sum for their relief. Furthermore, he made his own contribution. When the subscriptions did not reach the total anticipated, St. Vincent supplied the balance.

"On an occasion 200 livres[7] were wanting; he called the Procurator and the following dialogue ensued.

'How much money have you in the chest?'

'Just enough to feed the community for one day.'

'How much is that?'

'Fifty crowns.'[8]

'What! Is that all?'

---

[7] "The money value of the livre in 1600 was equivalent in purchasing power to 7½ francs (1907)." See note 38, Vol. I, page 13 in Pierre Coste, *The Life and Works of St. Vincent de Paul.* Westminster, Md., Newman, 1952.

[8] The crown was equal to two livres.

'Yes, that's all: I haven't another farthing.'

'Very well, then, bring it to me; I want it.'

The Procurator obeyed. But someone overheard the conversation and told one of the noblemen of the Association." One of them sent a purse of a thousand francs to Saint Lazare on the following day. [9]

Among the various types of evidence, referred to by Benedict XIV as bearing witness to heroic hope, is the joy that some have experienced at a sign that shows them that ᵈeath is near. We can illustrate this in St. Thérèse of Lisieux from a passage in her autobiography.

"During Lent last year I felt much better than ever and continued so until Holy Week, in spite of the fast which I observed in all its rigor. But in the early hours of Good Friday, Jesus gave me to hope that I should soon join Him in His beautiful Home . . . How sweet is this memory.

"I could not obtain permission to remain watching at the Altar of Repose throughout the Thursday night, and I returned to our cell at midnight. Scarcely was my head laid on the pillow when I felt a hot stream rise to my lips. I thought I was going to die, and my heart nearly broke with joy. But as I had already put out our lamp, I mortified my curiosity until the morning and slept in peace. At five o'clock, when it was time to get up, I remembered at once that I had some good news to learn, and going to the window I found, as I had expected, that our handkerchief was soaked with blood. Dearest Mother, what hope was mine! I was firmly convinced that on this anniversary of His Death, my Beloved had allowed me to hear His first call, like a sweet, distant murmer, heralding His joyful approach." [10]

The longing to die and be with God is one of what theologians speak of as God's mystic graces. This means that they are special gifts and cannot be obtained whenever we seek them. Ordinary graces, such as help in resisting temptation, are ours for the asking, but the mystic graces are special gifts which God bestows for reasons known to Him alone. This joy at the near approach of Death may be looked upon as the culminating point in the development of the theological virtue of hope. It is a proof, as Benedict XIV recognizes, that hope exists in the soul in an heroic degree.

---

[9] Op. cit. II, p. 396.

[10] Taylor's Translation, 1924, pp. 138-139. *Manuscript "C"*, pp. 5, left and right. The translation faithfully reproduces the original text.

CHAPTER V

Divine Charity

1. Divine Charity as Friendship Between God and Man

Charity is a theological virtue because it is concerned directly with God. It is an abiding habit by which we seek God above all created things, choosing Him by an act of the will. But as St. Thomas points out, it is something mutual. God loves us and wishes to give us all His Infinite Goodness that we are capable of receiving. And at the same time we love God, not because we want to get something from Him, but rather that we may give Him ourselves and all we may possess and consecrate to Him all our powers of being, doing, and suffering. Charity, therefore, is defined by St. Thomas Aquinas as a friendship between man and God.[1] Thus it says in Holy Scripture that Abraham was tempted, and being proved by many tribulations was made the friend of God. (Judith VIII:22).

When it comes to determining whether or not a candidate for canonization loves God purely and without any self-seeking, the ecclesiastical court demands facts that bear witness to the presence of truly heroic charity.

The reader will find in *Heroic Virtue* by Benedict XIV[2] an account of the "signs" that have been made use of by the auditors of the Rota[3] to determine this point.

We shall try to illustrate some of these signs from the autobiography and the letters of St. Thérèse of Lisieux. One that we have chosen is "similitude to God in such a manner as is competent to a creature in this life."[4] This concept is derived from a passage in the first Epistle of St. Peter. St. Peter writes that Christ "hath given us great and most precious

---

[1] *Summa Theologica*, 2.2. Q. XXIII, i.

[2] A portion of his treatise on the beatification and canonization of saints.

[3] The Rota at the present time is a tribunal consisting of a fixed number of Auditors for judging various causes. By a decree of Pius X, 1908, everything pertaining to the beatification and canonization of saints is referred to the Congregation of Sacred Rites. Codex Juris Canonici, 253, §3, note 2.

[4] Op. cit. I, p. 108.

promises: that by these you may be made partakers of the Divine Nature:
flying the concupiscence of that corruption which is in the world."[5]

2. Sinlessness as a Sign of Heroic Love of God

Habitual freedom from venial sin and the conquest of all imperfections is the necessary condition for truly partaking in the Divine
Nature: the Eternal Goodness. Thus one authority cited by Benedict
XIV speaks of a continuous uninterrupted course of innocency of life
for a long period of years on up to death, that so far transcends the
condition of man's nature "that it approaches closely to the essentially
changeless holiness of the Divine Nature" and "constitutes a man
perfect after the manner that our·Father in heaven is perfect."

Let us examine the life of St. Thérèse of Lisieux to find out how
early and in what way she tried to overcome all sins and imperfections
and so by innocence to become assimilated to the Divine Nature.

Before her mother's death, which occurred when Thérèse was 4
years and 8 months old, she was very actively engaged in correcting
her childish faults. Soon after they were committed she was intensely
sorry. There was a strong desire to go and confess to her mother and
a prompt resolution not to repeat the fault.

Her mother writes in a letter, quoted by Thérèse: "It is charming
to see her (Thérèse) run after me to confess her childish faults: Mamma,
I have pushed Celine; I slapped her once, but I'll not do it again."[6]

The combination of these three elements: sorrow, a desire to confess
and a firm resolution of amendment at so early an age is truly
extraordinary. It would be very difficult ordinarily to train a child to
react thus to every fault. Nor, if the attempt were partially successful,
would it be possible to elicit prompt spontaneous intense sorrow
by any training. We may well look upon this reaction as due to the
grace of God training a soul to cooperate with His guidance and pass
a whole lifetime without falling into any mortal sin, and perhaps even
to live without any or very few willful venial sins.

It has been said that "for a grown-up person to abstain throughout
his whole life, from every grievous sin whatever, of every description,

---

[5] *Heroic Virtue*, I, p. 108 (II Peter, i, 4.).
[6] Taylor's Translation (1920) p. 20. Manuscript page 7, right. See Chapter I of her
autobiography. St. Thérèse quotes from her mother's letters loaned to her for the
purpose by Pauline. See also hereon Stephane-Joseph Piat, O.F.M. *The Story of a
Family*, New York, Kenedy 1948, Ch. 9. *The Early Training of a Saint.*

is of all heroic acts the most heroic,"[7] and this was true of Thérèse (see below, page 118). Perhaps parental care and protection and teaching children to listen to the still small voice that urges to good would increase the heroism of innocence in our modern world.

The following passage refers probably to a period not long after her mother's death. It speaks explicitly of her ever-growing love of God and how she often offered her heart to God.

"As I grew older my love of God grew more and more. I offered my heart to Him, using the words my Mother taught me, and I tried very hard to please Him in all my actions, taking care never to offend Him."[8]

In this period before her mother's death she had already developed a habit of self-control that eliminated many imperfections.

"How happy I was at that age! I was beginning to enjoy life, and goodness itself seemed full of charms. Probably my character was the same as it is now, for even then I had great self-command, and made a practice of never complaining when my things were taken; even if I was unjustly accused, I preferred to keep silence. There was no merit in this, for I did it naturally."[9] But self-command comes by earnest practice. It is never a gift of nature. The passage is evidence that even at this early age the virtues of St. Thérèse were reaching the heroic level. For ease in doing good and the charms of goodness are the "facility" and "delight" that Benedict XIV demands for heroic virtue. But this does not mean that Thérèse had already attained to perfection in all things.

Did God use any human means to teach Thérèse the fundamental concepts of the spiritual life? The answer is yes. First, her mother taught her, as we have just seen, to offer her heart to Our Lord. After her mother's death and even before, it was Pauline who taught her, and her conduct in childhood was widely influenced by her.

Thérèse had permission to write notes to her sisters when they were on retreat. In one of these she wrote to Pauline: "How proud I am to be your sister! And your little girl, too, for it was you who taught me to love Jesus, to seek only Him."[10]

---

[7] Benedict XIV quoting F. Andrea Budrioli a Jesuit theologian. *Heroic Virtue*, I, p. 67.
[8] Taylor's Translation, 1924 edition, pp. 33-34. Manuscript, p. 16, left.
[9] Taylor's Translation, 1924, p. 26. Manuscript, p. 12, left. Passage commences on p. 11, right, continues to the left, then some sentences are cut out, and the last part is found below on p. 12, left.
[10] Collected Letters. Trans. by F. J. Sheed, New York. Sheed and Ward, 1949. Letter LXXXII, p. 123.

You can point to no period in which you can say of St. Thérèse that she then *commenced* to love God with all her heart and soul. She commenced to love Him as far as she could love Him when as a child God meant to her only something good, perhaps only vaguely distinguished from Pauline. When still very young and only able to say a word or two, she would lie still and think of Pauline. "When I was just learning to talk and Mamma asked: 'What are you thinking about?' my answer invariably was 'Pauline.' Sometimes I heard people saying that Pauline would be a nun, and without quite knowing what it meant, I thought: 'I will be a nun, too.' This is one of my first recollections and I have never changed my mind; so it was the example of this beloved sister, which, from the age of two, drew me to the Divine Spouse of the virgins."[11] And from that time on till the day of her death her love for her Divine Spouse ever increased.

3. *Unceasingly Seeking After God*

Benedict XIV mentions[12] as one of the signs of heroic charity to unceasingly seek after God: Seek ye the Lord and be strengthened: seek His Face forevermore. This was true of St. Thérèse, as we have seen, from the dawn of reason. Her letters and her autobiography show us that this seeking continued as long as she lived. Furthermore, this love of God and constant attempt to correct all her childish faults led to a cooperation with divine grace that, in turn, led to sinlessness of life. It will be well to quote here the words of Father Pichon, S. J., after hearing her general confession.

She tells us in her manuscript that they were the most consoling words she ever heard in all her life: "In the presence of the Good God, of the Holy Virgin and of all the Saints, I declare that you have never committed a single mortal sin."[13]

If one studies the autobiography of St. Thérèse with its citations from her mother's letters and her own letters, one has her own word and some objective evidence to support it for the conclusions.

  1. Moved by the love of Jesus which Pauline tried to awaken in her
      when Thérèse could only say a few words, it is evident that

---

[11]Taylor's Translation, 1924, pp. 21-22. Manuscript p. 6 right. Text develops all she owed to Pauline as her ideal. The development of this love for Christ can be followed on her letters to her sisters.

[12]*Heroic Virtue*, I, p. 108.

[13]Manuscript. 70 right, lines 13-14.

Thérèse not only commenced to love Our Lord at a very early age but also do her best to correct in herself everything displeasing to Christ.

2. At a very early age she commenced to manifest a sinlessness that approached the essentially changeless holiness of the Divine Nature, such as is required for the canonization of saints, and "constitutes a man perfect after the manner that our Father in heaven is perfect."

3. This process of drawing ever closer to the holiness of God, which Our Lord Himself asked of us, continued all throughout her life in which she never committed a single mortal sin.

4. The Span of Years Necessary for Heroic Sanctity

We may here raise an important question. As we have pointed out, there are only two ways to heroic sanctity: the way of innocence and the way of penance. When now one turns from a more or less sinful life and attains to heroic sanctity, how long must he persevere in heroic sanctity until death, in order to meet the Church's requisites for beatification and canonization?

Benedict XIV tells us that when he was Promoter of the Faith he heard some of the consultors assert "that it was necessary for the approbation of his virtues, that the servant of God should have lived heroically at least during the last ten years of his life, whether he was a servant of God, who before his conversion had been guilty of many sins, or who, free from grave offenses, had not lived heroically before."[14]

"In the cause of the venerable John Francis Regis ten years of the greatest toil and charitable zeal spent in apostolic missions were thought sufficient to justify a decree concerning his virtues."[15]

"When, however," says Benedict XIV, "I examined the grounds of this assertion, none were alleged: and I do not abandon the opinion which requires, indeed, a continuous heroicitry without defining anything about time. Therefore, when the case arises, it will be the duty of every one who has to give his vote in the cause, after considering the past career of the servant of God, to see whether, on the ground of length of time, during which he lived heroically, or on the ground of the nature of his actions, which he accomplished in a short

---

[14]*Heroic Virtue*, II, p. 402-3.
[15]Op. cit. II, 403.

space, he may be judged to have been a hero, and may be numbered among the saints who are worshipped* in the Church."[16]

5. Heroic Sanctity and Relapse Into Sin

But suppose that in the life of the candidate for canonization there came a relapse into mortal sin. This would be a serious difficulty for the demonstration of heroic sanctity. One might say that all would depend on the candidate's manner of life from his last mortal sin unto his death.

Benedict XIV takes into consideration the words of the prophet Ezechiel: "But if the wicked do penance . . . I will not remember his iniquities any more." But if a single fall prevented one who had been practicing heroic virtue from ever again rising to heroic virtue, God would be remembering his iniquities. Therefore, Benedict XIV arrives at this charitable conclusion: "It will not be sufficient that he who is converted to God after sins committed or that heroes who from time to time have fallen into sin, shall have shown signs of penance; but it seems necessary that they should have performed also so many and such exterior acts of Christian virtue and penance, that, as far as possible, it may be known, whether they have returned to that degree of holiness wherein they were once in the sight of the Church, or have been raised to a higher, or have remained in a lower degree."[17]

Perfect sorrow and a pure act of love for God on one's deathbed would suffice to gain heaven; but without some time lived in heroic virtue, such a person would scarcely be declared, by canonization, an outstanding example of the Church's heroes of sanctity.

To what extent can venial sin coexist with heroic virtue? "A venial sin is committed if with either perfect or imperfect knowledge and consent, one transgresses a law that does not oblige seriously; or, if with imperfect knowledge and consent, he violates a law that obliges gravely."[18]

---

*For non-Catholics who may not understand the use of this word in the Catholic Church we may say that worship (cultus religiosus) has three meanings in the Church: Cultus latriae or divine adoration which is given to God alone; Cultus duliae which is given to the saints. One may speak of this as worship but this word is seldom used at present to designate praying to or honoring the saints. The first meaning given to worship in Webster is courtesy or reverence paid to merit or worth; Cultus hyperduliae the special worship or honor given to the Blessed Virgin because of her divine maternity.

[16]Op. cit. II, p. 403.
[17]Op. cit. II, p. 407.
[18]Heribert Jone, O.F.M. Cap. Moral Theology. Westminster, Md., Newman, 1955, p.48.

Perfect consent implies full knowledge of what one is doing and a deliberate determination to do it.

Concerning deliberate venial sins Benedict XIV says: "If in the examination of a cause, when the question is concerning virtues in the heroic degree, it should appear that many sins, though venial, were frequently and deliberately committed, and no proofs were forthcoming of repentence and satisfaction, then in that case, it would be but reasonable to refrain from the approbation of those virtues."[19]

As examples of indeliberate venial sins one might mention inadequate control of sudden emotions, such as a flurry of anger, a drive to grumble and complain interiorly, a sharp word that slips out beyond our control. Of such semivoluntary venial sins, Benedict XIV points out that according to the Council of Trent it is impossible to avoid all venial sins throughout one's life unless one has a special privilege, such as that given the Blessed Virgin. And St. Augustine holds that no one except the Blessed Virgin had this privilege.[20] It would appear also that in the state of a purified soul which is like that of the Blessed in Heaven[21] the soul may go for long periods without a semivoluntary venial sin. But the virtues of a purified soul are not required for canonization.

Now as to heroic sanctity Benedict XIV writes: "If, indeed, some venial sins were committed inadvertently, and others with deliberation, and pains were subsequently taken to avoid them, and satisfaction made for them by works of piety, it would certainly seem hard and unreasonable to exclude a servant of God, illustrious for heroic acts, for that reason only from the honor of beatification and canonization."[22]

Sinlessness, as we pointed out, is the chief sign of heroic charity, for it means the union of the human will with the divine. And an act of charity is one by which the soul chooses God and rejects everything contrary to His will.

From the account here given, any earnest soul can be assured that with the grace of God he can certainly attain to heroic charity. Holy Mother Church in her wisdom makes no unreasonable demands. Heroic charity is yours if you will but make use of the torrent of grace that God will pour through your soul.

---

[19]Op. cit. II, p. 411.
[20]Op. cit. II, pp. 417. Council of Trent, Denzinger-Bannwart, 833.
[21]See above p. 17
[22]Op. cit. II, p. 410.

CHAPTER VI

Heroic Charity Towards Others

1. The Virtue of Charity

According to St. Thomas, what we love in any one with whom we come in contact is something good that we see in him. If we loved him only because we could get something good out of him that would be selfishness. But true charity is a love of friendship. But there is nothing truly good in any man except what is in God, for He is the Supreme Good and the source of all goodness found in creatures. So whether we love God or man, the object of our love is the goodness of God.

We might go on from this to point out that every creature capable of enjoying eternal beatitude in the vision of God for all eternity is our neighbor. We can say he is, at least potentially, our brother, for we are all united in the one mystical body, the Church, of which Christ is the head and we constitute the body.

When, however, we love anyone unselfishly it is because we see in him a reflection of the Divine Being. The reflection of the Divine Being is what we love and so in loving the creature we love God. St. Thomas writes: "The habit of charity extends itself not only to the love of God, but also to the love of our neighbor."[1] One and the same love extends itself both to God and man and constitutes not two virtues but one.

This is also the doctrine of Holy Scripture: "If any man say: I love God, and hateth his brother; he is a liar. For he that loveth not his brother whom he seeth, how can he love God whom he seeth not?"

"And this commandment we have from God, that he who loveth God love also his brother." (I John IV:20-21).

A word might here be said on hatred and antagonism. Hatred, to be a sin, must be a deliberate act of the will. There are some who, because another in various ways blocks their desires and checks their progress, or treats them with scorn or contempt, allow themselves to settle down to an abiding ill-will towards that person. This results in

---

[1] *Summa Theologica*, 2.2. Q. XXV, i.

their deliberately returning evil for evil and even wishing him every evil under the sun.

Of such as these St. John wrote: "He that hateth his brother is in darkness and walketh in darkness." (I John II:11). "Whosoever hateth his brother is a murderer. And you know that no murderer hath eternal life abiding in himself." (I John III:15).

On the other hand, many are very much troubled because they think a strong sensory antipathy is volitional hatred. You may say to yourself of another, "I can't bear to look at him. He gives me the shivers if I come near him." And such words are simple statements of fact and no sin *if you have never resolved to do any evil* to that person and especially if you pray that God will bless and prosper him.

2. *The Signs of Ordinary and Heroic Charity Towards Others*

Benedict XIV writes: "Among the signs of the ordinary love of one's neighbor are the spending of temporal goods in helping others, the undertaking of bodily labors in their behalf, the correcting of those in error, and bringing them back to the way of salvation, the forgiving of injuries, the caring for the salvation of souls and the wishing for them what we wish for ourselves."[2]

"And the signs and effects of heroic charity will be the doing the same whenever occasion offers, promptly, easily, expeditiously, pleasurably, not once or twice but frequently, and above all if the works which are done be difficult; so that from the whole collectively it may be inferred, that the man so working surpasses the ordinary mode of working in good men."[3]

It is quite certain that many a Little Sister of the Poor who has gone about her daily care for the poor in this manner, or the hospital sister tending the sick without murmur or any shadow of unkindness throughout the years of a long life, have gone to the judgment seat of Christ with at least one shining heroic virtue to their credit.

3. *The Poor Are Not Excluded from Heroic Liberality*

It is sometimes said that priests who have no personal fortune of their own or who are members of a religious community cannot manifest heroic charity by donations for the establishment of institutions to care for special needs. But St. Vincent de Paul points to the fact that there are exceptions. "His parents were hardworking and honorable tillers of the soil, who owned a good dwelling house and

---

[2] *Heroic Virtue*, I, 130.   [3] Idem, p. 131.

some acres of land."[4] Many a time in after life did the saint tell those
who showed him marks of esteem that he had tended cattle in his
youth, or even, quite bluntly, that he had been a common "swineherd."[5] His father started him on his education for the priesthood.
When he died, he asked the family in his will to see that his son's education was continued. St. Vincent, however, refused to allow the family
to sacrifice what they needed for themselves for his education. He
obtained money by taking charge of a little school and was such a good
teacher that it prospered, but not enough to support him entirely. He
was ordained with a big burden of debts.

It is incredible how vast were the sums he expended in well-
organized charity for all the woes of suffering humanity. A poor
swineherd became a center from which flowed a current that has
watered all the works of modern charity. Florence Nightingale is
responsible for the development of the trained nurses of our day. But
she went for her training to the Sisters of Charity founded by St.
Vincent de Paul.

It is also true that heroic charity in dispensing funds and care for
the sick can be organized on a large scale by a poor girl without
resources or influence of any kind. Mary Walsh was such a poor girl
doing laundry work for a wealthy family in New York. On her way to
work one sultry morning in the late summer of 1876, she saw a child
crying pitifully in the doorway of a cheap tenement. The child told
her that her mother was very sick and she did not know what to do.
The child led her to her mother. The poor woman seemed to be
dying. A dead child, just born, lay close beside her. Three frightened
children were huddled together in a corner.

Mary Walsh wrapped the dead child in a blanket and gave the sick
mother a sponge bath. There was nothing to eat in the apartment.
"This was a home only because it held a mother and her small family.
Otherwise it was a foul kennel of crushed humanity."[6]

What could she do? She promised the mother that she would be
back as soon as possible. She prayed as she went. She gathered
together her small savings and asked her friends to give for the love of
Jesus. She not only returned and gave the poor mother and her
children the first good meal that they had had in a long time, but
rehabilitated the home: fed them, cleaned the apartment, bought

[4] Pierre Coste, *The Life and Works of St. Vincent de Paul*. Westminster Md. 1952, I, 6.
[5] Op. cit., p. 8.
[6] Anne Cawley Boardman, *Such Love Is Seldom*, New York. Harper 1950, p. 3.

fresh bedding and clean clothes, paid the gas bill, buried the dead infant, got the husband out of jail, persuaded his employer to give the husband one more trial. "The result of her interest and hard work was lasting —the rehabilitation of a family that had been on the brink of disaster."[7]

In the meantime she had lost her own job. She said to herself: How many sick poor have no one to care for them! Why could I not work and get someone to work with me, live very simply and use our money and our toil to care for the sick poor.

The final result of the rehabilitation of this family, after many years of trial and hardship and working and begging for the poor, was the foundation of "The Dominican Sisters of the Sick Poor, a Group of Third Order Dominicans." There are now houses in New York, Ohio, Colorado, Michigan and Minnesota.

4. Heroic Forgiveness of Injuries

Love towards others and its heroicity may be demonstrated by forgiveness of injuries and extending the hand of fellowship to those who have injured us or worked against us. It is an easy way to heroic charity if we learn to make use of every such opportunity, promptly, easily, and with joy and delight.

Heroic examples of forgiveness were found in St. Maria Goretti and also in her mother, a wonderful peasant woman who trained her to be a saint and a martyr. St. Maria Goretti was stabbed to death when she was less than 12 years old, by a boy, Alessandro, because she would not yield to him. The priest who anointed her at the hospital asked her if she had forgiven her murderer. She answered, "Yes, I too, for the love of Jesus, forgive him," and then added the heroic words: "And I want him to be with me in Paradise." And then: "May God forgive him, because I already have forgiven him."[8]

Alessandro was sentenced to 30 years imprisonment, during the course of which he realized the heinousness of his crime and repented bitterly of what he had done to Maria. Discharged from prison many years later he went to see Marietta's mother on Christmas Eve. As soon as he begged pardon he was forgiven. Marietta's mother arranged that the two should receive communion side by side at the Midnight Mass, to let all the world know that Mamma Assunta had forgiven her child's murderer and all the world should do the same.[9]

---

[7] Op. cit., p. 4.
[8] See Marie Cecilia Buehrle, *Saint Maria Goretti*, Milwaukee, Bruce, 1950, p. 124.
[9] Pp. 150-151.

CHAPTER VII

Theological and Moral Virtues
in Psychotherapy

IF ONE WHO is a stranger to Christian thought reads these pages he will find it difficult to realize the fullness of their import. That will be particularly true of a psychiatrist who feels that he has every right to adjust the patient or lead him to adjust himself to his problems in life without regard to conventional concepts of morality. Such psychiatrists are not as numerous, it seems, today as some thirty to forty years ago.

1. *Psychiatric Treatment and the Moral Ideas of the Patient*

But it is not too much to say that the very concept of virtue has become hazy in the minds of a considerable number of people in our modern world. On the other hand, there are many belonging to various religious bodies who have fairly definite ideas about what is right and what is wrong; and it seems that their numbers are rapidly increasing.

And yet psychiatrists who have no religious convictions themselves are called upon to treat adolescents and adults who have problems that involve acute moral conflicts. Should not the psychiatrist at least know something about the religious attitude toward moral problems?

As we pass from the discussion of the theological virtues to the moral virtues it might be well to provide the reader with a simple outline of what a well-educated, religiously trained man of the world understands by virtue and a human being's obligation to practice it.

Let us first take the concept of the *natural moral virtues* which we are about to treat. Their development should commence in childhood and the parents should know what moral virtue is and seek to develop it in their children. They should have an end in view. That end—viewing life for the moment from a purely natural point of view—is to float the child in due season in the world about him and finally make the grown-up child a respectable self-supporting member of society. In the ordinary course of events the child will eventually have his own home and should be able to live in that home and contribute to its joy, peace and happiness. All this means that life for the child will be a series of moral problems on the way to being established in a home as a peaceful, useful member of a society in which all individuals and all homes live together in an abiding peace.

If now one asks how can the child be taught to solve the problems of life, the answer is that he must be led by kindly explanations to make use of his natural intelligence and reasoning power to adjust himself peacefully and harmoniously to each problem as it arises. He should learn that his moral ideal is to use reason and will-power in the light of ideals to control unwholesome emotions such as anger, hatred, laziness, and his drives to an unwholesome excess in satisfying his desires for food, drink and sex indulgence. The end in view will be to enable him to become a powerful personality capable of influencing others for good.

2. God and the Concept of Morality

We may now point out that there are two different groups of people who will agree with what we have said so far. One will be hazy about the concept of God as the source of the moral law. Or perhaps explicitly deny His existence. At the same time, those in this group will agree that it is reasonable for anyone in any stage of life to adjust his conduct so as to live harmoniously with others.

The second group is convinced of the existence of God as the source of all that is; and that the natural law written in the mind of every man imposes on him a moral obligation to keep the natural law. These will recognize that it is not only advantageous for them to live in harmony with others, but also that it is a sin against God to injure or cause trouble to those with whom they live; and a sin to waste life in the bewitching of trifling, instead of working hard from youth to old age to accomplish something worth while.

Reason sitting in judgment on conduct easily develops the importance of *prudence* in one's management of difficult situations. It also shows us the necessity of each one giving to others what one owes to them and of courts in which equal *justice under law* will be meted out to all. It also shows us the importance of patient endurance in all the difficult or painful situations in life so that prudence may aid us to go on from the moral battle to the triumph of *fortitude* and a new peace. And holding our natural goal in mind — a kind and helpful person in a home and an honorable member of society — we shall pass through life using the pleasures that come our way without abusing them in accordance with the laws that prudence lays down for us in the virtue of *temperance*.

The psychiatrist will find a number of patients who have more or less of this background as the basis of conduct. He would indeed be a rash therapist who would attempt to get it all out of the patient's mind because his own view of life did not tolerate any system of fixed morality.

3. Psychiatric Treatment of a Devout Christian

We come now to the patient who believes in God and is also a devout member of some religious body. It is here that the theological virtues loom more or less clearly above the horizon.

I would like now to ask the unbeliever, even though he is bitterly opposed to God and religion, to assume for the moment that God is the Eternal Omniscient and Almighty Wisdom, the Source and Origin of all that is, and that he has destined each and every member of the human race to enter on a pact of perfect and eternal friendship with Himself that will attain its fullness in the next life, when the soul will behold God as He is in Himself. From this assumption there flows the necessity of the existence of theological virtues.[1]

For it is perfectly clear that no man, by the mere light of natural reason alone, can direct himself to an end that transcends his natural powers of perception and attainment.[2] He must therefore be directed by God and aided by Him to attain what is naturally unattainable. As natural reason and will-power need natural virtues to attain the natural moral goal of an intellectual being, so any being, destined by God to a supernatural life and personal union with Him in a pact of perfect and eternal friendship and the vision of the Divine Essence in heaven, needs supernatural aids and virtues in order to know his end, seek it, and attain it. These virtues are known as *theological virtues* because they are immediately concerned with God and are produced

---

[1] St. Thomas, *Summa Theologica* 1.2. Q. LXII, i.

[2] Op. cit., 1.2. Q. LXII, i.

by God in the soul. According to Catholic belief, when a man is baptized he receives sanctifying grace. This grace produces a change in the essence of the soul in the form of an abiding quality akin to a habit.[3] Sanctifying grace will ripen in the course of life and when the soul enters heaven will burst into bloom so that the Divine Essence itself will act on the intellect without the intermediary of any concept, and man will see God face to face as He is.

With baptism one receives also the supernatural virtue of faith. St. Paul defines faith as "the substance of things to be hoped for, the evidence of things that appear not." (Hebrews XI:1). It makes us know God and speaks to us of our eternal life with Him and all that these truths involve. Furthermore, in illuminating the mind by faith the First Truth gives to the creature a special grace by which the evidence for "the things that appear not" is seen by the human mind in a special light and a man believes because God reveals.

Hope is an habitual craving of the human will to attain to that which the intellect knows by faith.[4]

Charity is a virtue which leads man to persevere in love and friendship with his Creator:[5] a state of spiritual matrimony, a pact of perfect and eternal friendship, the consecration of the human will to the will of God.

Suppose now that a psychiatrist is dealing with a devout Christian believer in whose mental problems moral difficulties loom largely in conscious and unconscious life; or suppose a psychologist has a problem of guidance in a juvenile delinquent which is rooted in an excessive and perhaps abnormal sexual drive. What should be their attitudes towards the devout believer's faith, even though they themselves think that all religion is a delusion?

I remember a psychiatric meeting in which a group of psychiatrists discussed this very problem. There were two attitudes:

1. The root of the patient's difficulty lies in his religion which is evidently a false set of ideas and may be conceived of as a delusional system. The psychiatrist's first problem therefore is to get rid of the patient's religion.

The other group said: "No! If you get rid of the patient's religion you will return him to his home with more problems than he had to

---

[3] 1.2. Q. CX, iii ad 3 um.
[4] *Summa Theologica*, 2.2. Q. XVIII, i.
[5] *Summa Theologica*, 2.2. XXIII, i.

start with. Therefore, you should adjust him to his difficulties in the light of his religious concepts."

4. A Psychiatrist Should Become Familiar with Fundamental Religious and Moral Concepts

In this work it will become apparent that religious ideals can be potent factors in the prevention of some mental disorders, and may even be used at times in therapy. The preservation and strengthening of virtue, both moral and theological, is a powerful factor in the preservation and establishment of sound mental health. Every psychiatrist should make himself familiar with fundamental concepts of religion and morality in devout believers. Unless he does so there will be many patients whom he can neither understand nor help.

A psychiatrist or psychologist with a violent antipathy to all things religious should raise the question in his own mind: Would I not become a better psychiatrist if I myself underwent a psychoanalysis or some form of mental readjustment?

Where moral problems are in the foreground, especially in a juvenile delinquent, one should have as the goal of therapy the adjustment of the patient to peace in his surroundings and settling down to making something worthwhile out of himself. One need not take up in a non-religious patient an ultimate philosophy of life.

But in dealing with the devout, a non-religious psychiatrist would do well, at the proper time, to call in the aid of the sympathetic clergyman or perhaps suggest that the patient see another psychiatrist. I say *at the proper time*. A psychologist in counseling should first give his mental and aptitude tests and study the adolescent thoroughly. He might use for some time bibliotherapy in which the patient by reading discovers what seems to him to be his own moral principles and ideals in life.[6] Where the patient commences to ask for help and advice, it is then the time to think of religious therapy, and seek the cooperation of a sympathetic priest.

The same is true of a psychiatrist dealing with a mental patient. He uses whatever techniques he thinks proper without ever attacking religion. He should become familiar with the ideals of the virtues if

---

[6] See hereon T. V. Moore, *The Nature and Treatment of Mental Disorders*, New York, Grune and Stratton, 2nd ed., 1951, chapter XIII. Bibliotherapy; and the *Driving Faces of Human Nature*, New York, Grune and Stratton, 1950, pp. 389-396. *Personal Mental Hygiene*, New York, 1944, pp. 178-181, 193-196, 221-224.

he accepts devout patients for therapy. And he, too, will sense a time in the treatment when the patient might be helped by a sympathetic clergyman of the patient's faith.

A psychiatrist should be familiar with fundamental moral and religious concepts. A non-Catholic psychiatrist should know that a devout Catholic gets his main help in the difficulties that confront him from what is termed the sacramental life of the Church. He knows that this help is supernatural and comes from God, and that it can never be replaced by any purely natural means such as the personal influence of others. In taking the history of a Catholic patient there might be a place for such questions as: Do you say morning and evening prayers? Do you go to Mass on Sundays? Do you receive Holy Communion once a year? Every month? Every week? Daily? Do you give some time to mental prayer daily? How often? Do you read the Holy Scriptures or books on the spiritual life daily? How often? What spiritual books do you like best? What devotional exercises do you practice?

The psychiatrist himself should ask these questions at a period in the treatment he selects, after there has been good rapport, or, as it is termed, good transfer, established with the patient. And even though he might not be a devout man himself, he should be a reasonable man and look upon the religious help that a devout patient gets from the practice of his religion as something that no psychiatrist should neglect in his treatment. By inquiry he should obtain the names of a number of good priests with practical common sense to whom people go for spiritual direction, try to know them personally, and from time to time ask their help in dealing with a devout patient.

The present period in the development of psychiatry has been spoken of as the *era of religion in psychiatry*. Efforts are being made by both psychiatrists and the clergy to find a ground of cooperation. This will be facilitated if all antagonisms are overcome on both sides. But beyond negative factors there must be something positive. Psychiatrists must become familiar with the ideals of the virtues and holy living, and priests must be given a general introduction to psychiatry.

CHAPTER VIII

Right Reason Applied to Moral Action

1. Charity, the Soul of All the Virtues

In the theological virtues we have just discussed, we have learned to know God's method of leading us to our end in eternal life. That discussion made known to us a great mystery: the mystery of God's love for man. He wants to establish a personal relationship with each and everyone of us. And that relationship is nothing less than a pact of eternal and perfect friendship between each human being and Himself. It means spiritual marriage between Christ, the Eternal Word made flesh, and every human being. Before that marriage can take place, the soul must attain to the heights of sanctity. From that truth you can deduce that you yourself, whoever you are and no matter how lowly may be your station in life, you are called to strive for and attain the highest sanctity of the saints. Our Lord offers you even now the pact of perfect and eternal friendship with Himself. How foolish it would be, how shameful, to refuse the friendship of the Lord, God Almighty.

From this you can see another truth: Charity, your love for God, is the soul of faith, hope and all the moral virtues. That means that you believe because you love God and crave to have God teach you all about your eternal life with Him in heaven. You hope because you love God and want to behold Him in heaven. Then coming to the moral virtues: You want to organize your life on earth according to the dictates of reason. You know that reasonable conduct is pleasing to God and keeps you from sin, so that you can be with God whom you will love for all eternity. And, therefore, you organize your whole life with prudence for the sake of God. By *justice* is meant a virtue by which we give to all men all that we owe them in any way. But we love all men because God loves them and we want to love God and all whom God loves, and far from withholding anything due, we would give even more!

By *fortitude* we endure patiently all the trials of life. We endure

52

them willingly because in that way we can give a proof of our love for God. The heavier the burden and the more painful a suffering may be, the more clearly do we manifest our love of God and prove its strength when we bear all with perfect patience, peace, joy, humility, and charity for the sake of God.

By *temperance* we thread our way through the snares of this world's pleasures without any misuse or abuse of the things that give delight in a world of temptation. And each renunciation, we make because we love God and reject the false good for Him Who is the Eternal Good, God Himself with Whom we have entered into a pact of perfect and eternal friendship.

In this way divine charity becomes the true life of every virtue. We have pictured it in its perfection but it will be long before you attain to that perfection. You will not always think with anything like full consciousness: I refuse, O Lord, this thing that is sinful or foolish or a worthless trifling because I love Thee and want to live in Thy love. Your pact of eternal friendship with the eternal good will sink into the background of consciousness; and you will battle in darkness.

But without our unconscious, abiding orientation to God and at times perhaps a fully conscious aspiration—For Thee, O Lord, for Thee alone —there is something wanting to virtue. It cannot rise to its perfection.[1]

One who bears the trials of life in stoic fortitude does something good; but it is something far below the burning love of Joyce Kilmer's Christian enthusiasm:

> Lord, Thou didst suffer more for me
> Than all the hosts of land and sea.
> So let me render render back again
> This millionth of Thy gift.   Amen.

2. Prudence and Its Importance

Prudence is a virtue of far-reaching importance in the spiritual life, and yet many works that treat of the spiritual life do not mention it by name. One can judge of its importance when we note that it is the function of prudence to direct the activity of the other moral virtues so that they may attain their end.[2] Though treatises on the spiritual

---

[1] St. Thomas Aquinas. *Summa Theologica*, 2.2. Q. XXIII, viii.

[2] *Summa Theologica*. 2.2. Q. XLVII, vi, Corpus. In the 5th article St. Thomas says prudence helps all virtues (therefore even the theological virtues) and works in all. Ad Secundum.

life give so little attention to it, in a process of canonization the prudence of the candidate is rigorously examined. A devout man devoid of prudence would not be canonized.

Benedict XIV thus defines prudence: "Right reason applied to moral action; and its object is whatever can be reduced to action, and falls under choice and reason."[3]

St. Thomas points out that prudence is good if skill is manifested in coordinating conduct to attain a *good* end; but if craftiness is used to attain an evil end, then such prudence is not good but false prudence. Furthermore, in order that prudence may be perfect the end sought must be directed ultimately to God. Pagan virtue that knows the good of the commonwealth and does not rise from the concept of nature to that of God is necessarily imperfect. The Christian who attains to true sanctity must refer all his actions to God and, without ever slipping back into a fully deliberate venial sin, he must tend with all his might to the highest Goodness and all his efforts must be directed ultimately to God.

It is in the moral virtues that our personal activity aided by divine grace is most productive of results. Personal effort and continual practice increase all natural virtues. Personal effort in the theological virtues does not increase them directly. For they are given and increased by God Himself. But fidelity to what God demands may merit that God in due season will increase our faith, hope and charity. Treating now of the Moral Virtues in which personal effort brings about directly their increase, let us speak directly to the reader.

3. Our Call to Heroic Virtue

In the first place you must remember that God wants you to attain to spiritual perfection; for Our Lord said to the common people in the sermon on the mount: "Be you therefore perfect, as also your heavenly Father is perfect." (Matthew V:48). This means that God wants you to attain to heroic sanctity. But does it mean that if I don't my failure would be in itself a mortal sin? No, the imperfections, venial sins and mortal sins that would keep you from perfection would sum up the extent of your responsibility, unless you had taken a vow to strive for perfection. Had you renounced all attempts to be perfect it would be at least venially sinful. But this does not mean that God does not want you to be perfect, for Our Lord has told us expressly

---

[3] *Heroic Virtue,* I, 136.

that He does. Be ye perfect as your heavenly Father is perfect. And Pius XI wrote: "All men of every condition, in whatever honorable walk of life they may be, can and ought to imitate that most perfect example of holiness placed before man by God, namely, Jesus Christ our Lord, and by God's grace arrive at the summit of all perfection."[4]

It would be well, therefore, to say to yourself, I want to be a saint and sanctity demands that the theological virtues should be of an heroic degree, that at least some of the moral virtues should be heroic, and all virtues should exist in a high degree. And so let us commence the study of the virtue of prudence, the queen of the moral virtues.

Benedict XIV points out the various fields in which the virtue of prudence may be exercised.

4. Prudence in the Control of Our Inner Life: Moods

There is an important field for *prudence* in the management of yourself; both in your inner life, and in your relations with other people.[5] If now you are going to attain prudence in a heroic or even a high degree you must use your intelligence to get perfect control of all undesirable emotions.

It has been said that the only way to control emotions is indirect, to turn the mind quickly to other things. But I think the reader will see that he will often be able to say: I am not going to keep on acting in that foolish emotional manner and simply banish anger, for instance, immediately. It will quickly simmer down as you go on about your business. It is also possible for a normal man, after some great sorrow, to bob up serenely on the next day and carry on his usual duties. Look at the matter from the point of view of prudence: some allow themselves to be overwhelmed because friends will come and be "so sorry for them." "Why," the prudent man will say, "should I behave in that foolish way any longer?" Practicing control of our inner emotions in this way by prudence we shall be able to acquire an habitual peace that will be hard to disturb. But the main factor in the development of emotional peace is a Eucharistic life in which mental prayer plays an important part. Peace invades one's life from the morning's

---

[4] Pius XI, *On Christian Marriage*, Nat. Cath. Welfare Conf. Ed. 1931, pp. 10-11.

[5] Benedict XIV calls this *monastic* prudence, not that it is confined to monks but rather because it concerns a single person's management of himself as distinguished from the individual managing a family or a city or an army in defense of his country against an invader.

Mass and Holy Communion and the time devoted to communing with
God spiritually in prayer. Many thousands could tell you that they
found it in that way. Perfect peace in all trials no matter how severe
is a sign of *heroic* sanctity. Do your part to maintain this peace always
and God will lift you to heroic sanctity and you will be the saint you
never thought you could possibly become. You should not allow
yourself to *want to be* canonized, for in this you might be seeking
yourself and not God. Very few of God's saints are canonized. Desire
above all to be united with God in that perfect union of mystic love in
which self is lost in the soul's union with God.

5. Prudence in Our Contacts With Others

Perfect peace and harmony in all interpersonal relations is also
demanded in a high degree, if not necessarily in an heroic degree, in
all those whom the Church beatifies or canonizes. Circumstances do
not always allow the manifestation of a high degree of peace with all
those with whom one comes in contact. Not every woman, for
instance, has a domineering inconsiderate husband who makes home
life a constant torture. But when this occurs it gives every one in the
family an opportunity to rise to truly heroic peace. I remember a
woman with two daughters and such a husband. In his most furious
outbreaks she maintained perfect interior and exterior peace. She
spoke to him only in a humble, kindly, affectionate manner. She
taught her two daughters to do likewise. If they all happened to be
saying the evening rosary and they heard the father coming, the
mother would simply say: "Finish the Rosary by yourselves, children."
And she would run to the door to meet him. The children were
taught to say their prayers before and after meals only if the father was
absent, for any manifestation of any kind of an act of religion made him
furious. The older daughter died of tuberculosis and I anointed her.
I think it must have been in his absence. That was now many years
ago. Some years later, the mother died. And it must have been the
mother's heroic peace that worked the miracle of his complete conversion shortly after she died. Then the father died, having received
all the sacraments of the Church. The remaining daughter was one of
those souls whom God cloisters in the wide open world. She lived
near a church and went to Mass and Holy Communion daily; she left
her house in the morning to go to work and came home to pray, till a
cancer that had developed made it impossible for her to work any

longer. Then having lived in peace she died in peace, and Christ received her with the angels and saints in the glory of eternal life.

Remember, good reader, that you too must attain a perfect interior peace, banishing all unworthy emotions of every kind and ever maintaining perfect peace in all your relations with others while you ever maintain that sublimity of soul that constantly tends with all its might to God, the final end of every human being.

6. Prudence and the Management of the Home

Prudence also concerns itself with the organization of the home. Our whole country is disturbed by the increase in juvenile delinquency. The most effective treatment of this evil would be adequate instruction in all high schools and colleges in the proper organization of a home. And then comes a principle that is largely lost sight of in our days: No home can be properly organized unless it becomes a school of the service of God. In this home the ideal of heroic sanctity must be well established in the parents and must dawn in the minds of the children as they come to the age of reason. There is a room and a place for psychiatrists and social workers who in due season and at the proper moment would make use of spiritual concepts in dealing with patients and clients who have the background that would enable them to understand religious ideals.

And so the organization of the home necessarily involves the development of a deeply spiritual life common to the whole family. The family as a family must have a spiritual life. It will not suffice to leave the spiritual life entirely to each individual as if he were a boarder in the household.[6]

But the home must also be organized so that all material needs are supplied and the children are prepared to enter life and take their place in the modern world. The appreciation of the value of education must be developed, and once some career has been chosen for a child the father must look into the proper lines of study to be followed. Prudence takes care not only of religious needs but also of the funda-

---

[6] One might see hereon the brief chapter in *The Home and its Inner Spiritual Life.* (by A Carthusian of Miraflores, Westminster, Md., 1952) on an "Ideal Father" based on R. W. Chambers; *Thomas More*, Westminster, Md. and Stephanie Joseph Piat. *The Story of a Family*, New York, Kenedy, 1948, and the *List of Readings for a Catholic Mother* in *The Life of Man with God* by T. V. Moore, New York, Harcourt Place, 1956, pp. 370-371.

mental material needs and the intellectual development of the
children.

A father or mother responsible for an ill-organized, dirty, slovenly
home would not possess prudence in a high degree. In a well-
organized home all the children are trained by word, but especially by
example in all the virtues. This training comes mainly from the
sanctity of the parents and the organic spiritual life of the family as a
family. This implies, when possible, daily Mass and Holy Communion,
the individual practice of mental prayer, the common and personal practice of holy reading. Many such homes exist. May they be multiplied!

7. *Prudence and the Family Consultation*

Benedict XIV says that when "Prudence" sits in judgment on
conduct, three things take place: (1) consultation; (2) decision; (3) the
final *command:* execute what has been determined.[7]

Consultation involves considering whether or not the end con-
templated is truly good and if so how it may be most easily attained.
The word "consultation" may be taken as meaning not only taking
stock of all "I know on the matter" but also in all important matters to
seek the advice of others.

St. Benedict in his *Rule* has a chapter, "Of Calling the Brethren to
Council," in which he says: As often as any important matters have to
be transacted in the monastery, let the abbot call together the whole
community, and himself declare what is the question to be settled.
And having heard the counsel of the brethren let him consider within
himself, and then do what he shall judge most expedient. We have said
that all should be called to council, because it is often to the younger
that the Lord revealeth what is best. But let the brethren give their
advice with all subjection and humility, and not presume stubbornly
to defend their own opinions.[8]

It might be well in every home to hold at times a family council
including younger children and ask the advice of all on anything
important, such as moving to another house or anything in which all
would be interested. St. Benedict seems to have drawn his ideal of an
abbot from that of a good father; and many things in his rule have
their counterparts in a well-organized home.

---

[7] Op. cit. *The Heroic Virtues,* I, 139.

[8] *The Rule of St. Benedict.* Trans. by D. Oswald Hunter Blair, Fort Augustus, Scotland.
Abbey Press, 1934, p. 25.

A good father will prudently organize life in his home so that all pray together, have their chief delight in being together, playing together, having vacations together and talking over together what is best to be done when any serious difficulties or problems arise. Then will the Holy Spirit Himself by His gift of counsel illumine the moral virtue of prudence and so He Himself will become the ultimate source that guides and develops the home.

CHAPTER IX

Heroism in the Service of God and Man

I

THE WORD "JUST" in scripture if often equivalent to holy, as
when the Lord promised Abraham that He would not destroy Sodom
if ten just men could be found there. (Genesis XVIII:32). But there
is another sense in which the word justice is used to designate *a virtue
which is manifested by a determination to give everyone his due.*[1]

In the broad sense justice means the possession of all the virtues and
becomes synonymous with holiness. But even in the restricted sense,
justice covers a wide range of conduct when we include under the
term all the virtues into which the definition can be divided or are
in some manner associated with it. Thus, then, we may divide justice
into two parts: (a) giving God His due and, (b) giving man his due.
Giving God His due then becomes the virtue of religion. Giving man
his due means that a man should recognize that his wife and children
have rights and he should never infringe upon these rights and should
be perfectly honest in all his dealings with others. All these things are
perfectly honest in all his dealings with others. All these things are
fundamental in the concept of that sanctity which is necessary for
beatification and canonization. An abundance of tender devotion is
not necessary for high sanctity; but strict observance of all the commandments is fundamental and its demonstration will always be
required in the canonical process of beatification and canonization.`

We can get a fuller comprehension of what will be investigated
under the name of justice in the canonical process by enumerating the
virtues that are looked upon as parts of justice. They are religion,
piety, observance, obedience, gratitude, vindication, truth, friendliness, affability and liberality. Thus, according to St. Thomas the ten
commandments "pertain to justice, as the first three acts of religion;
the fourth acts of piety; and the other six acts of ordinary justice;

---

[1] See St. Thomas, *Summa Theologica* 2.2. Q. LVIII, i.

60

which applies to parties who are equal."[2] Let us now develop the concepts of the various virtues that in some manner pertain to *justice*.

II

Religion is a virtue by which we give God His due. This is done when we worship Him by prayer and sacrifice.[3] In our day the Holy Sacrifice of the Mass has taken the place of the sacrifice of animals under the old law. The minimum we can do is be present at Holy Mass on Sundays. But those who go to Mass and receive Holy Communion daily possess the virtue of religion in a high degree. When this is done constantly and in spite of great difficulty, one may rise even to the heroic degree of the virtue of religion. Thus, when one who may be unable to go to early morning Mass, goes to work year after year and fasts till noon and then goes out, hears Mass, takes a hurried breakfast and returns to work and does this every day, he may be said to practice the virtue of religion in an heroic degree. And by no means few are those who do this. They are the salt of the earth.

III

According to St. Thomas, just as it belongs to *religion* to show devotion to God, it pertains to *piety* to manifest devotion to one's parents and to one's fatherland and to all one's relatives and to all one's friends and fellow citizens.[4] A man who did not love and help his parents, or who did not love his country and support her in the hour of danger would not qualify for canonization.

IV

Observance is a virtue by which one shows respect and honor to persons in a position of authority. St. Paul established this as a fundamental Christian duty: "Let every soul be subject to the higher powers. For there is no power but from God: and those that are ordained of God. Render therefore to all men their dues. Tribute to whom tribute is due: custom to whom custom; fear to whom fear: honor to whom honor." (Romans XIII:1 and 7).

"Husbands, love your wives, as Christ also loved the Church, and delivered Himself up for it." (Eph. V:25). "Wives, be subject to your husbands as it behooveth in the Lord. Children, obey your parents in

---

[2] *Summa Theologica* 2.2. Q. CXXII, vi.

[3] See St. Thomas, 2.2. Q. LXXXI.

[4] *Summa Theologica*, 2.2. Q. CI, i.

all things: for this is well pleasing to the Lord. Fathers provoke not your children to indignation, lest they be discouraged." (Col. III: 18-21). "Being of one mind one towards another . . . To no man rendering evil for evil. Providing good things . . . If it be possible, as much as is in you, have peace with all men." (Romans XII:16-18).

It is readily seen that all this is impossible, unless Divine Charity gives life to all the virtues. And all this is demanded of everyone that is beatified or canonized. No troublemaker in the state, the family, the place of employment, or in the world at large can qualify for sanctity.

V

Obedience is a virtue demanded by the very structure of society. St. Thomas derives its concept from the world of nature. Modifying his terminology we may say that he calls attention to the fact that the motion of the planets in our solar system is due to their exact, prompt, unswerving obedience to the law of gravity. And in the living world all the organs of a living being obediently cooperate to supply the needs experienced by the organism itself. They work in obedient harmony for the welfare of the whole. Then calling attention to the gradations of authority in the state, he says: As in the divinely instituted natural order itself the lower things in nature are by necessity subject to the direction of the higher, so also in human affairs, by natural and divine law, subjects are bound to obey their superiors.[5]

This holds in all ranks of political government and in the family and also in any large or small business enterprise. One should learn something about obedience from the solar system. Our will should be so trained to obey that lawful obedience will be as prompt and effective as the law of gravity in nature. In any group of which you are a member, let prompt, cheerful and wholehearted obedient cooperation be the law of your life. Of course, you will frankly and humbly express your opinion when matters are being discussed. But when a plan of action has been determined, your cooperation should be as perfect as the movements of the planets in the solar system.

We may consider a passage from the rule of St. Benedict as giving expression to some qualities necessary in heroic obedience.

"Such as these, therefore, leaving immediately their own occupations

---

[5] *Summa Theologica* 2.2. Q. CIV, 1.

and forsaking their will, with their hands disengaged, and leaving unfinished what they are about, with the speedy step of obedience follow by their deeds the voice of him who commands; and so as it were at the same instant the bidding of the master and the perfect fulfillment of the disciple are joined together in the swiftness of the fear of God by those who are moved with the desire of attaining eternal life. But this very obedience will then only be acceptable to God and sweet to men, if what is commanded be done not fearfully, tardily, nor coldly, nor with murmuring, nor with an answer, shewing unwillingness: for the obedience which is given to superiors is given to God."[6]

VI

Gratitude is a virtue by which we duly acknowledge and do not forget the gifts, help and kindness we have received from others, both great and little. It should be expressed sincerely in words and we should show honor and respect to our benefactor and if the tables are turned we should give help to our benefactor in his hour of need.

Our acknowledgement of all we owe to God, the Infinite Good from Whom all blessings flow, is manifested by the virtue of *religion* and consists in adoration, love and service in doing His will by keeping the commandments.

The acknowledgement we make to our parents by love and obedience and helpfulness is termed *piety*.

The honor and respect we give to persons in authority for what we receive from them was known by the term *observantia* (observance).

The rendering of thanks to special benefactors for their gifts and helps of all kind is the virtue of *gratitude*.

A vivid picture of what the gratitude of a saint was is found in the life of St. Vincent de Paul.

"If a benefactor met with financial losses, he was always ready to return his gifts: 'What a happiness,' he said one day, 'to impoverish ourselves to assist those who have done us a kindness.' He had more than one opportunity of experiencing this happiness. 'I beseech you,' he wrote to a former benefactor, 'to make use of our property as if it were your own; we are ready to sell everything we have for you, even our very chalices; by doing so we shall only be carrying out what is laid down by the holy canons, and that is to return to our founder in his hour of need what he gave us in his days of prosperity. I am telling you

---

[6] Rule of St. Benedict. Op. cit., Ch. V.

this, sir, not out of politeness but before God and I feel it in the depth
of my heart.' "[7]

VII

Vindication as a virtue is an established good habit by which one in
authority inflicts penalties not out of a spirit of revenge but in an
attempt to lead the wrongdoer back into the paths of justice.

As St. Thomas says, when vindication in a human person is revenge,
it belongs to hatred and not to the virtue of justice.[8]

A judge of the present day in a criminal court is, however, limited
by the written law and the decision of the jury. A wise and virtuous
judge, nevertheless, might in various ways check the unreasonable
zeal of a prosecuting attorney to secure a conviction at all costs and
block the presentation of evidence that would prove the innocence of
the defendant. Lawyers also can practice this virtue in vindicating the
rights of the innocent.

Vindication in the sense of St. Thomas should also be an outstanding
virtue in every father and mother. Sometimes parents become
insensed against a child and want to punish him, and do punish him
severely. Punishments so inflicted may be directed at hurting the
child out of a desire for revenge and are not really imposed after due
reflection to make sure that the child will mend his ways and do better.
St. Anselm's way was to have what he termed a cheerful conversation
with the unruly boy, for in that way he found that he more easily led
him along the path of good conduct. The scriptural passage "spare
the rod and spoil the child" should not be interpreted so as to mean
that whipping is the only method of correction. No, it forbids that
parents should always let children go their own way without *any*
attempt to guide their conduct and develop their virtues. As St.
Thomas says, vindication is a mean between two vices: "one by excess,
namely the sin of cruelty or ferocity, which goes beyond due bounds in
punishing; the other, however, is a vice which consists in a defect as
when one is unduly remiss in punishment."[9]

But if one sees that a whipping will only make things worse, it
would be a mistake to whip. A parent might very well then attempt
to see what might be accomplished by kindly explanations and talking

---

[7] Pierre Coste, C. M., *The Life and Works of Saint Vincent de Paul.* Westminster, Md.,
1952, III, 315-316.

[8] St. Thomas, 2.2. Q. CVIII, i. Corpus.

[9] *Summa Theologica*, 2.2. Q. CVIII, ii ad 3um.

things over. I remember my mother would, at times, talk things over and explain my conduct till I would cry. And thinking it all over on going out, I once felt that I would rather have a licking any day.

But there is another sense of *vindication:* "to support or maintain as true or correct, against denial, censure, or objections" (Webster). In this sense all those who in public or in private vindicate the revealed doctrine of God and the teaching of His Church practice the virtue of vindication, a part of justice, which attempts to secure for God from men all that which is His due.[10]

Benedict XIV cites one of the authorities (Sacchus) who says that in the process of canonization the Roman courts do not examine the life of the candidate for the due practice of absolutely all the virtues but examines "with reference to the circumstances and condition of each, those acts only which belong to his rank and condition, whether a subject of a prelate, who ought to have at heart in a special manner the practice of distributive justice."[11]

But with regard to the second type of vindication, the defense of the teaching of the Church, any layman, not isolated from all contact with others, will have abundant opportunity to practice the virtue of vindication, if he obeys the injunction of St. Peter: "Sanctify the Lord Christ in your hearts, being ready always to satisfy everyone that asketh you a reason of that hope which is in you." (I Peter III:15).

VIII

In his discussion of *truth,* St. Thomas deals with lying, simulation and hypocrisy. As far as telling the truth, whether by words or signs, is concerned, all know well the sinfulness of falsely representing to others what is in their mind.

But there is another sense which might be included here: pretending to be what one is not; to be a person "wellborn" in the wealthier or noble members of society, whereas one's parents were poor and in no way distinguished. There is a tendency, felt very strongly by some who are of what the world calls of "low birth" to hide their humble origins, in spite of the fact that Christ was born in a stable. They rise by education or wealth or some great success to the better classes and pretend to be what they are not.

---

[10] In a process of canonization such attempts are usually presented as evidence of the candidate's *faith.*

[11] *Heroic Virtue,* I, pp. 157-158.

Among the canonized, St. Vincent de Paul felt this tendency keenly. But he conquered it completely, put himself to shame and in that way practiced in an heroic degree the virtue of truth. He would not yield to pretense.

There are many incidents in the life of St. Vincent de Paul which makes it perfectly clear that he would not allow himself to sail under false colors. His work in later years led him to enlist the nobility in the service of the poor. Lest his contact with the noble and wealthy might lead others to think that he was of noble or wealthy parentage, he repeatedly said in the presence of others: As a boy, I was only an ordinary swineherd and my parents were peasants.[12]

"About 1628, when the Congregation consisted of seven or eight priests residing in the Collège des Bons-Enfants, he knelt before them all and publicly confessed the gravest sins of his past life."[13]

One day one of his country relatives came to see him. St. Vincent felt ashamed to have him presented to others as his relative and told the porter to bring him to his own room. But immediately seeing through his attempt to appear as what he was not, he hastened down to the door and presented the boy as one of his relatives.

IX

Friendliness and affability are treated by St. Thomas as one and the same virtue.[14]

The necessity of friendship arises from the fact that men ordinarily live together in social intercourse with one another. Now in order that all may go on smoothly it is necessary that there should be a mutual friendly love between all members of society.[15] The necessity of this friendly love between all affects the relation between those in higher authority and their subjects. A story is told of St. Louis IX, King of France (1214-1270). A woman who apparently had an anticlerical complex waited to give him a piece of her mind when he would leave his royal palace. So she ran up to him when he appeared and commenced to scold: A pretty kind of king you are! Why don't you attend to the business of the kingdom? It is nothing but the Franciscans this

---

[12]Pierre Coste, *The Life and Works of Saint Vincent de Paul.* Westminster, Md., Newman, 1952, III, p. 295.
[13]Op. cit., p. 297.
[14]2.2. Q. CXIV *Concerning friendship.*
[15]2.2. Q. CXIV, ii, ad primum.

and the Dominicans that, and so she went on. When St. Louis got a chance to say a word, he spoke to her with great patience and kindness: My dear lady, what you say is true. I am not fit to be a king. But God made me king and I try to do the best I can. Come to me at any time when I can help you and I will attend to your problems as if they were my own.[16]

This story of a saint illustrates the Thomistic concept of friendship when it has risen to a heroic degree. In spite of insults friendliness is not disturbed and the royal help is proffered whenever it will be needed. It also illustrates the Roman concept of affability. The affable man is easy of access; anyone can speak to him at any time. Insult is not returned for insult. No matter what happens, he is always kind and friendly.

Cardinal Newman was a violinist and that led him to a beautiful concept of intimate friendship. A friend, he says in one of his sermons, plays upon the soul of his friend, as a violinist upon his violin, and brings forth all its hidden melodies. In this sense Christ alone can be a true friend. But we should have the ideal before us in all friendly contacts with others. But to carry it out effectively, every friend must pray and work to be another Christ in his own interior life and in his dealings with others.[17]

The reader may have found this chapter somewhat prosaic, but if he will stop to think, it throws an important light on what a saint is and on what the reader should become. Too often, sanctity is understood as concerned mainly with visions and revelations. But neither visions nor revelations are demanded of a candidate for beatification and canonization, but kindness is.

X

Among the virtues that follow in the train of justice is *repentance or sorrow for sin* committed. This sorrow leads to a firm resolution never to offend God again and a desire to make satisfaction as far as we can for the offense we have given to Him Who is Infinite Goodness and Eternal Love. Sorrow for sin is not only an act of contrition but it is

---

[16] I read the story years ago in a Spanish work on the lives of the saints, which is no longer available to me.

[17] Liberality is the last of the "parts" of justice enumerated by St. Thomas. The reader might consult pp. 43 where we show that even the poor can rise to heroism in liberality, not only in the sense of the widows mite but by the measure of what they actually do and give in the course of a lifetime.

also something that abides within us as long as we live. For should there ever come a time when we are no longer sorry for having offended God, our sin would return. But works of reparation could be terminated after various periods according to the gravity of the sin.[18]

It is evident from this that repentence is a virtue that constitutes a part of justice because it concerns giving to God what is due because of sin.

Let us now attempt to illustrate it from the example of Mary Magdalen at the feet of Christ in the banquet hall of Simon, the Pharisee.

If we ask ourselves the question: What led Mary Magdalen into the dining hall of Simon the Pharisee? the answer comes that again and again she had hung on his words as he was speaking to the people. What was the burden of Christ's teaching? At one end as it were, we may say it is expressed by the words: "The time is accomplished and the kingdom of God is at hand: Repent and believe the Gospel." (Mark I:15). And then it ascended to the heights: "Be you therefore perfect as also your heavenly Father is perfect." (Matthew V:48). And then he said, no doubt on more than one occasion: "I am the good Shepherd: and I know mine and mine know Me—and I lay down My life for My sheep." (John X:14-15).

Through such words Mary Magdalen came to realize that Christ truly loved every sinful soul. And then there dawned a light and she asked: Can He possibly love even me? She pondered over such words as: "Therefore doth the Father love Me: because I lay down My life that I may take it up again" (John X:17). And the true light that enlighteneth every man who cometh into the world illumined her mind one day when she heard Christ say: "I and the Father are one." (John X:30). And there came to her intimations of something she could not understand and still felt it must be so: Christ is indeed one with the Eternal Father and is truly God and at the same time truly man. And then something like thunder rumbled in the depths of her mind the words of the Ten Commandments and she realized how she had sinned against the love of Christ. By this time it was already true what Christ was to say of her: she loved much.

The beauty of our Lord's personality and His love for her had already been made known to her by grace after grace received while

---

[18]*Summa Theologica* 3, Q. LXXXIV, viii.

listening to His words. And there came over her a sorrow for sin that flowed from a realization of the divinity of Jesus and that her sins were a long list of serious rejections of the love of God, one with the love of Jesus, the Shepherd Who was going to lay down His life for her salvation, Who was God and man, born into this world that he might gain the love of sinners like herself.

In the days of Jerusalem before the fall, there was a custom of public banquets to which any could go and stand listening to the conversation of the invited guests. These banquets performed some of the functions of a good newspaper with its editorials in our days.

Mary went to listen. Moved by a sudden impulse she stepped forward and "standing behind at Christ's feet she began to wash his feet with her tears and wiped them with the hair of her head and kissed his feet and anointed them with the ointment."[19]

She remained motionless and in silence at Christ's feet as He spoke to Simon of the cold reception He had met in his house in which the ordinary courtesies of the day had been conspicuous by their absence. She realized as He spoke that our Lord's own words were indeed true. Never would he cast out anyone who came to Him. And then he pronounced over her those words of absolution: "Thy sins are forgiven thee"; and after a pause: "Thy faith hath made thee safe. Go in peace." "Safe" she repeated to herself and there welled up a resolution within her: I will never sin again: a resolution of such a character that once made it is never broken. There are indeed some conversions like that of St. Paul. They are absolutely permanent and one who takes them never turns back. The resolution of Mary Magdalen, as she left the dining hall of Simon the Pharisee, was one of these immutable determinations.

Can it be said Mary Magdalen washing our Lord's feet with her tears and drying them with the hair of her head is merely an example of a woman in a violent state of emotion?

To understand this problem we must hold clearly in mind what St. Thomas Aquinas says about the nature of emotional experience. If any one experiences delight it must be because he becomes aware in some way of something that is good or pleasant. If anyone experiences grief or pain, it must be because he becomes aware of something that is evil or in some way hurts. But the good and the evil are objects of

---

[19]Luke vii, 38. The word *standing* suggests that the table and couches on which the guests reclined were elevated above the floor.

human desire. Human desires are of two kinds, those due to the perception of sensory goods and those due to the perception of goods that intellect alone can understand. We thus have in man two types of emotions, those that are reactions to sensory perceptions and those that are due to intellectual insights.[20] The simpler pleasant perceptions of sensations like the odor of a rose are termed the sensory feelings; but man is a unit being of body and soul in whom sensory perceptions are seldom devoid of intellectual insights. Hence his complex emotional states. A starving man might get suddenly angry like a dog if anyone tried to snatch away what he was eating, without any noticeable admixture of intellectual insight. Frequently, however, our emotions are mingled with sensory and intellectual processes. The bodily resonance is the same in both sensory and intellectual insights. Thus the tears of St. Peter when he went out and wept bitterly were a bodily resonance due to the intellectual insight into what Christ had been to him and how he had been false to his Master in the hour of our Savior's need.

Returning now to St. Mary Magdalen we can see that a series of events must have transpired before she went into the dining hall of Simon the Pharisee and washed the feet of Christ. These events familiarized her with the teaching of Christ and perhaps, as suggested above, not only with the beauty of His character but also with His divine personality. She had gone through a process of spiritual development in which she had come to realize the true meaning of sin: infidelity to the love of God Whom she knew in Jesus Christ, the promised Messiah, true God and true man, the Good Shepherd who knows each one of His sheep and calleth each by name. She had come to feel that Christ was indeed calling her by name and she had to go to Him.

Now it is clear that all these things intellect alone can understand. To them, all our sense organs are blind.

We might point out here that the concept of St. Thomas about the two kinds of emotions, sensory and intellectual,[21] enables us to understand better what is meant by sensible devotion and spiritual consolation.

In sensible devotion much is due to a purely natural heightened emotivity. Some people can shed tears at will and any feeling of

---

[20]*Summa Theologica* 1, 2. Q. XXXI iv and v and Q. XXXV, 1.
[21]*Summa Theologica*, 1, 2. Q XXXI, iv and v, Q XXXV, i.

delight is likely to cause tears of joy. Any new undertaking flows over easily into enthusiasm. But there is no deep intellectual insight into the spiritual meaning of what has been undertaken. Any project demands some intellectual activity. One cannot see, hear, taste, smell or touch a "project." One who understands, let us say, "a spiritual life," must at least know intellectually that he is undertaking something, but he may have very little understanding and appreciation of what he is undertaking and yet bubble over with enthusiasm. These are those who have purely natural sensory devotion. They are those of whom our Lord spoke in the parable of the sower: "some fell upon stony ground, where they had not much earth: and they sprung up immediately, because they had no deepness of earth. And when the sun was up they were scorched, and because they had not root they withered away." (Matthew XIII:5-6).

Sometimes this joy and enthusiasm which have no natural reason for their existence are graces that God gives to the soul. They are then accompanied by a desire to learn more of God and the spiritual life by mental prayer and holy reading.

Spiritual consolations are something quite different: St. Teresa of Avila says that what she calls consolations come from the Prayer of Quiet.[22]

In the Prayer of Quiet, God gives the soul a quasi-perceptual realization of his presence which absorbs the mind to such a degree that the body, entirely of itself, tends to remain still and motionless. Furthermore, during this quiet, quasi-perceptual realization of the Divine Presence, the soul glows rather than flames with the love of God. It is clear that the basis of the prayer of quiet is God's action on the intellect, filling it with a knowing of His Presence; and an inspiration of the will awakening the personal consecration of the soul to God which is Divine Charity, the love of the soul for God—which is not God but which attains to Him even in this life.

We have pointed out that the love of Mary Magdalen for Christ was of such a character that through the action of divine grace accompanied by her own total cooperation, her conversion became something permanent like that of St. Paul.

How can we attain to such a permanent conversion. It has been said that true conversions in and outside the Church are always

---

[22]See *Interior Castle* IV, ii. Peer's trans. II, 236.

sudden, permanent, and to something better. I would replace the word true by some. For conversions that last and develop and in the course of their growth become so immovable that the soul never returns to the fleshpots of Egypt are also true conversions. Much here is a matter of mere terminology.

But how am I to make my turning to God permanent? The Thomistic distinction between sensory and intellectual emotions and the example of Mary Magdalen point the way.

My enthusiasm for progress in the spiritual life must become deeply rooted in living intellectual ideals. My knowledge of Christ must grow. I must become intimately acquainted with His personality. I must *know* His love for me. And out of this knowledge of Who Christ is and of His love for me there must grow a supreme, overwhelming sorrow born of this knowledge. A sorrow in which I know myself as I am and that Christ is my Eternal Lover. In this sorrow there will not be a shadow of anxiety nor a trace of despair, but something that will lead me to the feet of Christ, knowing full well that when I come to Him, He will not cast me out.

In all this I need but follow Mary Magdalen. *She* hung upon His words. This I do in my life of prayer and holy reading. I live in His presence and listen to what He has to say. And one day His call will bring me to His feet. Have Mercy on me, O Lord, according to Thy great mercy. And I shall hear the words: Thy sins are forgiven thee. Thy faith hath made thee safe. Go in peace. Thou art mine forever more!

Some psychiatrists, whose mental gaze is fixed on the states of sorrow and anxiety with which they are familiar in mental hospitals, look upon all sorrow for sin as pathological. They might well ponder on this analysis of the sorrow of Mary Magdalen at the feet of Christ.

CHAPTER X

The Fortitude of the Saints

1. What is Fortitude?

The natural virtue of Christian fortitude is ordinarily concerned with the more or less strenuous difficulties of life. But human difficulties present a hard task in two ways: some arrive from allurements to the pleasures of life and settling down to a sinful enjoyment of them in idle ease. Others frighten the weak minded away from doing the good that they clearly perceive. The virtue of temperance restrains the allurements to sin and the virtue of fortitude awakens us to fight vigorously against everything that makes it hard to do the good we clearly see.

Fortitude in one sense is a certain firmness of mind that keeps us from wavering. When the difficulties are of a minor character they need no special virtue to conquer them. For every good habit, to be a virtue, must have a stability of its own.

When, however, the difficulties are extreme, dealing with them becomes such a battle with dangers and persistent endurance of labor that it passes over to a special virtue and is given the name of fortitude. It is a mean between two extremes, a moderation of unreasonable rashness and the conquest of undue fearfulness. Every soldier who "goes over the top" has to overcome fear. But it is reasonable to do so and go over with the rest. I remember the instance of one soldier near where I was in the First World War who went out on his own without orders and with his rifle alone walked up to a trench of German soldiers and commenced firing at them only to fall at once pierced by many bullets. Such an act was not an act of the virtue of fortitude because it was unreasonable.

But fortitude is concerned specifically in *reasonably* facing death in war in defense of a good cause. But it extends itself to any circumstances in which the fear of death is involved.[1] Thus a priest who stays

---

[1] *Summa Theologica* 2.2. CXXIII, v.

at his post to care for the sick and gives them the last sacraments in a dangerous pestilence or a nurse who serves on a ward of infectious diseases practices the virtue of fortitude.

Furthermore, when one courageously puts up with difficulties and dangers that do not involve death, he may be said to practice fortitude in an extended sense of the word (secundum quid).[2] It is only in this sense that most people have an opportunity to practice fortitude. And only in this sense can the virtue of fortitude be demonstrated in the lives of many saints.

Thus, Benedict XIV gives its definition: "Fortitude may be defined to be a habit, or virtue strengthening the mind to do or suffer those things which are agreeable to right reason."[3] And again more fully: "Acts of Christian fortitude, in so far as it is a common virtue,[4] consist in attempting difficult things agreeably to right reason and from a supernatural motive, and this in all matters whether of precept or counsel. But acts of heroic fortitude will consist in attempting the same things easily, readily, and with pleasure, even at the risk of the loss of all one's goods, or of life itself. Again to suffer patiently for God's sake evils, calamities, and pains are acts of common Christian fortitude; but acts of heroic Christian fortitude . . . consist in bearing cheerfully and readily, for God's sake, these and the like things, or even much more difficult ones, and death itself, when there is need of it."[5]

2. Fortitude as a Gift of the Holy Spirit[6]

The virtues are good habits enabling man to follow the dictates of reason. "They perfect man according as he is by nature moved by reason in all his interior and exterior activity."[7] Did man exist in pure nature and had he no destiny to a supernatural life with God in eternity, he could attain natural happiness on earth by the light of reason alone. The modern world, to a large extent, has lost sight of man's supernatural destiny. It does not see in the guidance of man anything more than reason. In many child guidance centers of our

---

[2] *Summa Theologica* 2.2. CXXIII, iv, Ad primum.
[3] *Heroic Virtue*, I, p. 167.
[4] All virtues contain an element of fortitude in an extended sense. But Benedict XIV seems to be contrasting here fortitude in the extended sense in its non-heroic and heroic stages.
[5] *Heroic Virtue*, I, pp. 171-172.
[6] *Summa Theologica*, 1.2 Q. LXVIII. i, corpus.
[7] *St. Thomas*, loc. cit.

day, neither psychiatrists nor social workers pay any attention at all
to the guidance of children to their supernatural end. It is not good
form to introduce the concept of guidance towards an eternal end in
many a child guidance center. And, all too often, guidance conflicts
with the natural moral law.

But man has a life in heaven for which he must prepare himself if he
is ever to attain eternal glory and happiness.

"Now this is eternal life: that they may know Thee, the only true
God and Jesus Christ Whom Thou hast sent. .

"Father, I will that where I am, they also, whom Thou hast given
Me, may be with Me; that they may see My glory, which Thou hast
given Me, because Thou hast loved Me before the creation of the
world." (John XVII:3 and 24).

But man by the light of reason alone cannot find his way to eternal
life. Therefore, over and above the virtues "it is necessary that there
should be in man certain perfections, higher (than the virtues), by
means of which he receives a tendency to allow himself to be moved by
God"[8] to his eternal end in heaven, even as by the virtues he is directed
to natural happiness on earth. And these higher "perfections" are
called the *gifts of the Holy Spirit.*

Among the gifts there is fortitude which arises from the direct action
of the Holy Spirit on the mind of man leading him to put up with every
difficulty, little or great, and guiding him in the darkness and trials of
life so that he will not lose his way, but get over every obstacle that
blocks the road to eternal life with God. This transcends the powers of
all nature. Thus, St. Thomas writes: "Fortitude demands a certain
stability of mind." This same stability is required in carrying out good
works and enduring evils, especially when great difficulties are involved
in fulfilling these duties.

Man, moreover, can have this same stability, in regard to doing good
and putting up with evils, in a way that is proper and connatural to
himself so that he does not weaken in doing good on account of any
difficulty or the effort involved in its accomplishment, or having to
suffer any injury.

But the mind of man is moved still further by the Holy Spirit, that
he may carry on to the end what he has once commenced, and get over
every danger that threatens. This, however, exceeds the powers of

---

[8] See *Heroic Virtue*, II, 172 ff.

human nature."[9] That is when the end for which man is striving is a supernatural end. It is for such ends that the gifts of the Holy Spirit are *necessary*.[10]

3. The Religious Life and the Gifts of the Holy Spirit

Let us now consider the concept of the gift of fortitude in relation to one's entering a religious life and undertaking by the vows to strive for spiritual perfection *usque ad finem vitae* even to the end of life. Can that striving be commenced and maintained steadfastly to the end by strength of will and the natural virtues or is it necessary that the member of a religious order should be guided and sustained by the gifts of the Holy Spirit?

We have just seen that according to St. Thomas the virtues are able to guide man to that natural perfection that accords with the dignity of an intellectual being. But they do not suffice to guide man to attain the supernatural ideals, in virtue of which he becomes perfect as his Heavenly Father is perfect and so can enter eternal life in heaven. But the essence of the religious life is to renounce all things earthly by the vows of poverty, chastity and obedience and so stretch forward to the union of the soul with God in eternal life. That principle answers the question; but we may get a fuller picture from a chapter in St. Paul's epistle to the Philippians. (Phil. III:7 ff).

There he tells us of his life before his conversion as a Hebrew of the Hebrews. He had attained to a knowledge of the Law and a respected position in the eyes of all his people. As a Hebrew he could ask no more. But then Christ called him. He was baptized and Christ led him alone into Arabia and made known to him by revelation the whole theology of the New Law, and sent him forth to "carry His name before the Gentiles." We cannot in our day appreciate the sacrifice this change meant to a Hebrew of the Hebrews in the Apostolic age.

St. Paul thus refers to the renunciation he made at the call of Christ: "The things that were gain for me, the same have I counted loss for Christ. Furthermore, I count all things to be but loss for the excellent knowledge of Jesus Christ, my Lord: for whom I have suffered the loss of all things and count them as dung that I may gain Christ."

---

[9] 2.2 CXXXIX, i, Corpus.
[10] 1.2. Q. LXVIII, ii, Corpus.

The joy of youth with which a young man or a young woman approaches the altar to pronounce his vows does not always rise to the enthusiasm that rings in the words of St. Paul. But in essence the vows of poverty, chastity and obedience demand the selfsame renunciation. The one who thus consecrates his life to God will never know the joy, the delight, the satisfaction of a great duty well done of the man or woman who establishes a home that is truly a school of the service of God: The years of pure and beautiful affection surrounded by happy children and the joy of teaching them to know and love God.

And then there will come the "burden of the day and its heat." The school sister, with her prosaic life, perhaps, in a little town, one morning like another in the school room, correcting exercises in the afternoon and preparing lessons. When the vacation comes, there is the summer school and preparation for degrees. And later on teaching in the community's own summer school; and so on throughout life. There are indeed the cheerful daily recreations and perhaps, at times, such a thing as a picnic with the children. But things that the world sets so much stress on as a summer of travel, the theatre, opera, social functions, there is nothing of that.

Perhaps the hospital sister has an even harder life with the daily care of patients, who are not patient, on the wards.

A priest in a parish will tell you that he scarcely has time to say his office. Anyone who takes a kindly interest in the problems and troubles of others will soon learn that his late afternoons and evenings are filled with appointments for weeks in advance

In our day no one has the perils of waters, perils of robbers, perils from his own nation, perils from the Gentiles, perils in the city, perils in the wilderness and perils from false brethren that enlivened the years of St. Paul. But a good priest who does all the good he can do is likely to be often as busy as Christ and His Apostles who did not even have time to eat.

4. The Gift of Fortitude and the Perpetuation of Religious Communities

If one studies the history of religious communities in the Church they become one of the most remarkable phenomena in all history. The original and prototype of all was that of Christ and the College of Apostles. A common purse sufficed for the needs of all. This was continued and developed in the first community of Christians in Jerusalem. "And the multitude of believers had but one heart and one soul. Neither did anyone say that aught of the things which he possessed was his own: but all things were common to them." (Acts IV:32).

In the meantime another root of the religious life sprouted. Certain ones took a vow or promise of celibacy that they might live more easily a devout life of prayer *in their own homes*. St. Paul in no way condemning marriage held up to both sexes the principle that the practice of a devout life in virginity was even more noble than Christian marriage: "He that is without a wife is solicitous for the things that belong to the Lord: how he may please God. But he that is with a wife is solicitous for the things of the world: how he may please his wife. And he is divided."

"And the unmarried woman and the virgin thinketh on the things of the Lord: that she may be holy both in body and in spirit. But she that is married thinketh on the things of the world: how she may please her husband." (I Cor. VII:32-34).

From the times of St. Paul on there was a body of celibates, men and women, in the Church of whom the Church was proud. "Those who had decided to live a celibate life and to carry out various kinds of renunciation soon obtained a special position in the Church, even when they did not enter the ranks of the clergy."[11] They were known as *continentes* and were both men and women and at first lived in their own homes. But as early as the year 270 when St. Anthony of the desert, at about 19 years of age, was preparing to learn all things to enter on the life of a hermit, there was a much respected group of holy virgins to whom he could entrust the care of his little sister. It became a natural thing for the *continentes* living in their own homes to live together and organize various works of charity.[12]

St. Benedict of Nursia (480?-543) established in about 529 a monastery on the summit of Monte Cassino from which monasteries of men and women were founded all over Europe. The monastic infirmary developed into the only hospital of the region and the school for novices became the only school for many miles around; and the rule of St. Benedict the only law of the region. Thousands upon thousands became monks and nuns renouncing all that they possessed and lived

[11]*History of the Primitive Church* by Jules Lebreton and Jaques Zeiller, New York, MacMillan, 1947, II, p. 1105-1106.
[12]St. Athanasius, *The Life of St. Anthony*, transl. by Robert J. Meyer, Westminster, Md. Newman, 1950.

a common life of perfect chastity under obedience to an abbot or abbess.

In 1957 there were in the United States 49,725 priests, including 19,244 in religious orders, 9,300 lay brothers and 162,657 nuns. Looking upon secular priests as living a celibate life under obedience to their bishops and all religious priests as living a life of poverty, chastity and obedience, this is a vast army, in the United States alone, who continue the life the Apostles led under Jesus Christ, our Lord. But this same religious life is led all over the known world. Religious poverty with common ownership of property, and life under obedience to a superior, has continued in the Church for nearly 2000 years. All other attempts to establish a common life can point to no such universality in time and place; and most often such attempts die out after a short existence, as, for instance, Brook Farm in Massachusetts from 1841 to 1847.

The reason for such failures is the fact that the natural virtue of fortitude is incapable of the common endurance in all members of a group that is necessary for such a movement to carry on for centuries leading souls to perfect sanctity and in the end eternal life.

Great works have been carried out by religious communities in the past, and are being carried out now and will be until the end of time. And in all active orders there is the daily grind which we have just illustrated.

But behind these activities there is something that comes from the action of the Holy Spirit on the soul: something that is the very essence of the life in enclosed contemplative orders. St. Paul speaks of this when he says that he gave up all things "that I may know Him, and the power of His resurrection, and the fellowship of His sufferings: being made conformable to His death."

"If by any means I may attain to the resurrection which is from the dead.

"Not as though I had already attained, or were already perfect: but I follow after, if I may by any means apprehend. . . .

"Forgetting the things that are behind and stretching forth myself to those that are before.

"I press towards the mark of the prize of the supernal vocation of God in Christ Jesus." (Phil. III:10-14).

All this is essentially the life of God's laborers in this our day. It is surprising to what heights the Eucharistic life can develop and mingle with the work of the day, and make endurance possible.

One nun speaks of "dreading to leave the chapel in the morning when the 'intimacy with Christ was so wonderful and return to the unhappy world' even though she knows that Christ will accompany her every step she takes. When school is out 'I almost run home to get to Him in the Blessed Sacrament even though He has been with me all day long. It is a case of carrying Himself to Himself to adore and praise Him on the way and in the tabernacle.' "[13]

In all this we see not mere strength of will and the natural virtue of fortitude but the living picture of the gift of the Holy Spirit giving strength to the soul through its life in time while on its way to the perfect union with God in eternity.

-----

[13]T. V. Moore, *The Life of Man with God.* New York, Harcourt Brace, 1956, p. 232.

Chapter XI

Human Reason and the Pleasures of Life

1. The Law of Temperance

Man differs from brute animals in as much as he is capable of governing his conduct by reason. At the same time the world in which man lives has many more attractions than the brute world. Furthermore, even from the point of view of mere nature, man has an end: the development of his personality in accordance with the ideal of a perfect man. But man's sensory cravings are not all in accordance with the ideal of a perfect man and he experiences powerful urges contrary to this ideal.

Man, therefore, needs an habitual way of acting that when a powerful urge drives him to act contrary to that ideal, he may promptly reject the urge and obey the dictates of reason. These habitual ways of acting are the moral virtues. Temperance is specifically concerned with the pleasures of sense and mainly those concerned with eating, drinking and the propagation of the species. Men must do these things in order to live and that the human race may continue to exist. He must have a rule in order to so enjoy them that the dignity of his personality may be maintained.

St. Thomas formulates this rule as follows: Temperance looks upon the necessities of this life as the rule for enjoying its pleasures. Man should use the pleasant things of this life only in so far as the necessity of this life demands.[1]

St. Ignatius made this law of temperance the fundamental principle of his whole spirituality. "Man is created that he may praise the Lord our God and show Him reverence and praise Him, and by so acting save his own soul.

"The other things on the face of the earth are created for man to help in the attainment of his end on account of which he was created.

"Hence it follows that man should use these things only in so far as

---

[1] 2.2. Q. CXLI, vi, Corpus.

they help him to his end and should withdraw himself from them in so far as they hinder him in attaining his end."[2]

But all this refers to renouncing pleasures but not to the infliction of punishment. Thus St. Paul says: "I chastise my body and bring it into subjection: lest perhaps when I have preached to others, I myself should become a castaway." (I Cor. IX:27). Furthermore, all the canonized saints have been outstanding in their practice of bodily austerities.

It would seem at first sight that the infliction of pain would have nothing to do with temperance which seeks a mean between extremes. But St. Thomas includes abstinence, fasting, chastity, and virginity under the virtue of temperance. The justification for this he gives when he treats of fasting.

2. The Motives of Self-Denial

An act is virtuous when it is ordered by reason for the attainment of something that is truly good. This is true of fasting. It is undertaken mainly on account of three things.

1. To repress the concupiscence of the flesh: whence St. Paul says: "in watchings, in fastings, in chastity, in knowledge, in longsuffering" (II Cor. VI:5-6), for chastity is preserved by fasting.

2. That the mind may be more freely elevated to the contemplation of higher things. Hence, Daniel said that after three weeks of fasting, he received the revelation from God. (Daniel X:2 ff.).

3. To make satisfaction for sins. "Be converted to me with all your heart, in fasting and in weeping and in mourning." (Joel II:12).

3. Reasonableness in Self-Denial

Taking fasting as signifying all manner of penitential acts involving some kind of self-inflicted pain we may say that the *heroic temperance* of the saints is to be sought in what they renounced for God and in the manner of their "fasting."

But it is well to point out here that in the matter of self-inflicted penance that temperance has to establish a mean, dictated by prudence. Benedict XIV writes thus: "After the Apostle Paul, in his epistle to the Romans (Romans XII:1), had said, 'I beseech you therefore, brethren, that you present your bodies a living sacrifice,

---

[2] *Exercitia Spiritualia S. P. Ignatii De Loyola,* edited by R. P. Joanne Roothan. Augsburg, 1887, pp. 44-57.

holy pleasing to God,' he adds, 'your reasonable service', and the Interlinear Gloss on this passage explains it: 'With discretion, without being excessive.' Lyra explains the word 'reasonable' to mean that the body is to be mortified, but in such a manner as to preserve it and keep it free from vice; since the body ought not to be rendered unable to fulfill its own duties and offices."[3]

On the other hand it must be shown that the candidate for canonization was truly earnest in the practice of self-denial. Benedict XIV quotes the following passage from Sacchus: "In the acts of the Servants of God, not martyrs, which are examined into for their canonization, those in whom the desire of mortifying the flesh is not apparent, are not to be regarded. Accordingly, with respect to these, it is not unreasonable to suspect their sanctity, nor is it, I think, allowable to propose their worship or veneration in the Church of God. For with the exception of martyrs, the Church venerates and gives the sanction of her authority to the sanctity of those only whom she finds to have been zealous in the mortification of the flesh and senses."[4]

Since, therefore, for canonization all the moral virtues must be present in a high degree and some in a heroic degree, (see above, page 14) what is the minimum self-denial demanded and what is excessive?

4. The Example of Christ

Some light is thrown on the problem of self-denial by the example of Our Lord. He has shown us that some self-denial is not only lawful but also important in our spiritual life. We may be unable to do all that He did, but does that justify us in doing nothing?

Our Lord was about to commence the great work He came into the world to accomplish. At the same time He was about to be tempted by the devil. He needed no fast to obtain light and strength for His work, nor to meet the attack of Satan—but we do. And, therefore, He set us an example of how to prepare for the work that is before us and to resist the attacks of Satan. And because this is true, Holy Mother Church very early in her career instituted the Lenten fast.

But we live in a pleasure loving world that invites us to share its pleasures. Even good men say to us: "Come along. Be reasonable.

---

[3] Benedict XIV, *Heroic Virtue*, I, pp. 553-554.
[4] *Heroic Virtue*, I, p. 322.

The good things of life are to be enjoyed. Don't go to extremes. Steer your way along the mean path between unreasonable asceticism and the whirlpool of vice." All this is true in the abstract. But in the concrete: what are the extremes and what is the mean between them?

Let us look for a moment at the problem from the point of view of pure philosophy. Aristotle indeed tells us that virtue is a mean between two extremes. But he says it is not an arithmetical mean, that is, a point equally distant from the two extremes. For he says in order to escape the whirlpool of Charybdis one must steer well over toward the Rock Scylla. In like manner, from a purely natural point of view, we cannot escape shipwreck in life without earnest hard self-denial, rowing with might and main. for the whirlpool of Charybdis is a powerful torrent and we must keep well away from it to escape it.

If now we ask what is the Christian tradition, we have the example of Christ just mentioned, and need go no further. But St. Paul represents also the ideals and practices of early Christianity. "Everyone that striveth for the mastery refraineth himself from all things . . . I therefore so run, not as at an uncertainty: I so fight, not as one beating the air. But I chastise my body and bring it into subjection: lest perhaps, when I have preached to others, I myself should become a castaway." (I Cor. IX:25-27).

One might develop the treatment of the early Christian practice of self-denial. Suffice it to mention their weekly fasting.

"In the first two centuries, the faithful fasted twice a week, on Wednesdays, perhaps in reparation for the treason of Judas, and on Fridays in memory of the Passion. . . . These fasts consisted in abstinence from all food and even all drink until the ninth hour, that is, until the middle of the afternoon."[5]

5. Are Works of Penance Necessary for Salvation?

We may now raise the question: Is mortification of the flesh and body by such things as fasting, midnight rising, hair shirts, the discipline and kindred penitential exercises, necessary in order to enter eternal life?

The answer of Benedict XIV is that if we except fasts and other things commanded by the Church, it is not necessary in order to a

---

[5] *The History of the Primitive Church* by Jules Lebreton and Jacques Zeller, New York, MacMillan, 1949, I, p. 508.

man's attaining eternal salvation.[6] "Yet," he says, "In order to reach the summit of Christian perfection it is necessary."[7]

The question then naturally arises: what practices of self-denial and to what extent must I practice them, if I am going to attain my desire and reach the summit of Christian perfection?

6. *The Upper Limit of Self-Denial is Not the Same for All*

In coming to this conclusion Benedict XIV makes an important distinction between virtue itself and practices by which virtue is acquired. There is, for instance, no upper limit for faith, hope, charity or any virtue. One cannot be told to be virtuous up to a certain limit. But granted that self-denial is a helpful means in turning us from vice to virtue we cannot deny ourselves everything. We have to eat to live and so some limit must be set to fasting. Then a big powerful man doing heavy labor must eat more to live and work than a small girl employed as a stenographer.

St. Augustine felt keenly the difficulty one experiences in setting limits to desire in eating and drinking.

"I strive daily against concupiscence in eating and drinking. For it is not of such a nature that I can settle on cutting it off once for all, and never touching it afterwards as I could of concubinage. The bridle of the throat then is to be held attempered between slackness and stiffness. And who is he, O Lord, who is not some whit transported beyond the limits of necessity?"[8]

Eating and drinking is neither a vice nor a virtue. But its regulation by temperance becomes a virtue and by lack of regulation becomes the vice of gluttony. There is no such thing in self-denial as one and the same standard level to which all must rise.

No one should practice acts of self-denial that interfere with the performance of one's duties. Nor should any one in a religious community take it upon himself to practice openly works of self-denial that are not prescribed by the rule, and so fall into the vice of singularity.[9] Works of self-denial beyond the rule of one's order or

---

[6] *Heroic Virtue*, Trans. by Fathers of the Oratory, London, Thomas Richardson, 1850, I, p. 337.

[7] Op. cit. 1, 338.

[8] *The Confessions of Saint Augustine*, Trans. by E. B. Pusey, Mount Vernon, New York, Peter Pauper Press (no date), p. 216.

[9] *Heroic Virtue*, I, p. 353.

congregation should not be undertaken without permission of the superior or the spiritual director or both.

We have noted the passage in St. Paul which appeals to Christians to live an earnest life of self-denial but with discretion. After St. Paul, in his epistle to the Romans, XII, 1, had said: "I beseech you, therefore, brethren, that you present your bodies a living sacrifice, holy pleasing to God," he adds: "your reasonable service." Reasonable here means: deny yourself with discretion.

But we must not rationalize to escape the burden of self-denial and reason away a vigorous, but reasonable and wholesome earnest life of self-denial. If we do we cannot attain to the perfect spiritual life to which all are called in the sense of Our Lord's words: Be you therefore perfect as also your heavenly Father is perfect. That means heroic sanctity. Benedict XIV says: A stop should be put to the cause of a servant of God who is a confessor, if proof is wanting of a due and fit amount of bodily austerities during his life.[10]

7. *What Forms of Self-Denial Must I Practice?*

What then must *I* do? Perhaps the best I can do in the line of suggestions is to digest for the reader the fourth chapter in the rule of St. Benedict.

First of all keep the Ten Commandments and honor all men.

Then deny yourself in order to follow Christ.

Chastise the body and seek not after delicate living.

Love fasting and relieve the poor, practising the spiritual and corporal works of mercy; and prefer nothing to the love of Christ.

Not to give way to anger and exert good control over all your emotions.

Pray for your enemies in the love of Christ.

Make peace with an adversary before the setting of the sun.

And never despair of the mercy of God.

All this may be summarized in the injunction: Give up your own will and devote yourself completely to doing the will of God.

But many of the words in this digest are general and do not give me specific instructions. How much, for instance, shall I fast? What bodily penances must I choose?

In speaking of the measure of drink, St. Benedict quotes St. Paul and says: "Everyone hath his proper gift from God, one after this

---

[10] *Heroic Virtue*, I, p. 351; see also p. 349.

measure and another after that." (I Cor. VII:7). You may take that as meaning that you should consider the whole matter honestly in the Divine Presence. Go before the Lord in the Blessed Sacrament and pray and think. As you do so various practises of self-denial will come before your mind: I should make great sacrifices to keep this or that commandment. I could be helpful to others were I mindful of such and such spiritual works of mercy. Perhaps like the early Christians I could fast on Wednesdays to make reparation for the treason of Judas and on Fridays in memory of Our Lord's Passion. And so on; but don't resolve too much at first but only a few resolutions. Later on you can add.

8. Function of a Spiritual Director and the Rule of a Religious Community

Benedict XIV warns against settling this matter then by ourselves. We must seek the approval of our spiritual director and do neither more or less than he approves. For those in a religious community the basic practices of self-denial are defined by the rule. Benedict XIV says that in the process of canonization of members of any conventual institution: "It must be proved that they have not omitted those austerities which are prescribed by rule."[11]

9. More Prayer Does Not Make Up For Neglect of Self-Denial

This is evident from the rule that for heroic sanctity one cannot be lacking in any virtue. The various practices of self-denial are not in themselves virtues; but their regulation by reason is a virtue.[12]

It sometimes happens that a latent quietism lurks in the mind of one who gives up or is lax in the practice of self-denial.

The following propositions of Molinos were condemned:

"*The three ways:* purgative, illuminative and unitive, are a supreme absurdity as spoken of in mystical writings. There is only one way, namely, the internal."[13]

"The voluntary cross of mortification is a heavy burden and fruitless and is therefore to be laid aside."[14]

The true attitude is expressed by Benedict XIV: "If mortification of the flesh is wanting, it is difficult to open the way to contemplation."

---

[11]*Heroic Virtue,* I, p. 370.
[12]St. Thomas, 2.2. CXLVI, i.
[13]Denzinger-Bannwart, 1246.
[14]Denzinger-Bannwart, 1258.

He then quotes Gerson: "Bodily afflictions exalt the mind to what is high and great, while they nerve and brace it against falling lower . . . It will . . . astonish me if he who makes a practice of drawing back from the hardships of fasting and other mortifications, is not found to be far off from exalted contemplation.[15]

Perhaps the ultimate reason for this is that there is a close interconnection between the virtues. If faith is weak, hope is not strong, if faith and hope are far from what they should be, the fires of charity burn low. If faith, hope and charity remain on the level of first beginnings, there is no earnest self-denial, and little interest in progress in mental prayer, and the graces to make this progress are denied.

Then we must consider that it is the clean of heart who see God. Self-denial appeals to the Mercy of God, sins are promptly forgiven and the soul is pure in His sight. The King of Nineveh heard of the preaching of Jonas; "and he rose up out of his throne and cast away his robe from him and was clothed with sack cloth and sat in ashes" (Jonas III:6) and all the people did penance with him. "And God saw their works, that they were turned from their evil way" and had mercy upon them.

He who leads an earnest life of penance is ever washing out the little sins he daily commits and so remains clean of heart and becomes holy. Therefore, in contemplative prayer he easily rises to the veiled vision of the Majesty on high.

With good reason then does Benedict XIV quote one authority as saying: "Those in whom the desire of mortifying the flesh is not apparent, are not to be regarded. Accordingly with respect to these it is not unreasonable to suspect their sanctity."[16]

As a good holy life approaches the level of heroic sanctity the soul is no longer separated from God by occasional mortal sins nor even by fully deliberate venial sins. It is held back by semi-deliberate faults which might be termed trifling were it not that they hinder so great a good.

The root of our sluggishness is in the cold soil where love is lacking. Beg God to increase your charity, "Whatever good work thou beginnest to do, beg of God with most earnest prayer to perfect."[17] And He will.

---

[15]*Heroic Virtue*, I, p. 351.
[16] Ibid., I, p. 322.
[17]Prologue to Rule of St. Benedict.

CHAPTER XII

Heroic Sanctity and our Life of Prayer

1. The Life of a Good Christian is a Life of Prayer

Every good Christian should not only pray but lead a life of prayer. As a matter of fact this is done even by the laity of the laboring classes far more extensively than is ordinarily realized. Let me present the example of a pipefitter.

He rises every morning at six, because he wants to hear Mass and receive Holy Communion before he must be at his job and commence work. After washing and dressing there is time to read a little from the imitation of Christ or the account given in his Missal of the saint or feast of the day. During Holy Mass he tries to recall this early morning reading.

Once in the church he renews his Morning Offering in the presence of the Blessed Sacrament. "During the Holy Sacrifice," he writes, "I pray for various intentions, for the Church suffering not only in purgatory, but here on this globe, in those countries that say there 'is no God,' and the State is master of the destiny of man; for peace, if it be God's will to lift the scourge of war; for all those in their last agony, or in danger of dying impenitent, that they may recall God's love and mercy; for those who are weighted by the cares of the world; for those whose life has become dull and meaningless that they may taste and see that the Lord is sweet and feel the joy of life; for the grace of final perseverance."

After communion he makes his thanksgiving. The church with all its familiar furnishings disappears and he feels himself "in a vast measureless void, surrounded by the Infinite Immensity of the Blessed Trinity. But the minute hand moves quickly on and severs this sweet bond. The world, the flesh and the devil are waiting outside; but I have fortified myself with charity and He is a seal upon my heart."

In a little bit he is on the job; but lives with Christ while he works. If he flips a drop of hot solder on his hand it is something to offer to Christ. If he has to carry heavy iron piping he thinks of Christ carrying His cross.

Finally the hard day's work is done. He goes at once to a Catholic church near his room. He carries with him a book by St. Alphonsus Liguori for visits to the Blessed Sacrament. But sometimes he is too tired to read and simply kneels before Our Lord offering Him the fatigue of the day's work.

Then back to his room he washes up and for a little while reads a book on the theory of the work he does on the job. After supper he goes to a Catholic library and reads till it closes. He then goes back to his room. You cannot say that it is a lonely room for He lives with Christ. At 10:30 he says Compline and reads something from St. Francis de Sales. "In case I can't focus on one thing, I'll switch off the light and say the Rosary. Mary never fails to tuck me in: *Mater amabilis*."[1]

The spontaneous personal prayer of this pipefitter, for all the faithful that suffer and are in need of help, is that which every one of the faithful should do as members of the mystical body of Christ. Such prayers ascending to heaven from vast numbers of the faithful on earth are a powerful influence in the conversion of those who lead a sinful life and also of unbelievers who know not God.

On Ash Wednesday the Church reads from the second chapter of the prophet Joel where God tells him to ask for special prayer and fasting for the conversion of His people.

"Now, therefore, saith the Lord: be converted to Me with all your heart, in fasting and in weeping and in mourning.

"And rend your hearts and not your garments, and turn to the Lord your God: for He is gracious and merciful, patient and rich in mercy...

"Blow the trumpet in Sion: sanctify a fast, call a solemn assembly...

"Between the porch and the altar, the priests the Lord's ministers shall weep and shall say: spare O Lord, spare Thy people, and give not Thy inheritance to reproach." (Joel II:12-17).

These words express the spirit of the Church in the holy season of Lent, praying for the sins of the faithful.

We may say of the faithful what St. Benedict said of monks: that their lives should have about them something of a Lenten character. Thus many good Catholics go to Holy Mass and Communion daily during Lent. How much more would be accomplished in their own souls and the souls of others if they did this all through the year?

---

[1] T. V. Moore, *The Life of Man with God.* New York. Harcourt Brace, 1956, pp. 4-7.

Let us now take the example of one who held the position of supreme authority in the Church: St. Pius V (1504-1572). He looked upon it as a special duty of a Supreme Pontiff that, for the welfare of the faithful, his life should always have about it something of a Lenten character.

Benedict XIV draws the following picture of it based on the account of the Bollandists.[2] Pius V, realizing that prayer is of great assistance to all, determined to make his daily life a constant prayer for the sanctification of the faithful. And so he rose at dawn to commence his prayers for the faithful. So deep became his prayer that when anyone came to him about a matter of importance they had to give a little tug on his sleeve to arouse him. When he rose to leave his prayer he was still not fully conscious of his surroundings. He could only give a fragmentary answer to questions, so deeply had he entered into divine contemplation.

Furthermore, he even went so far as to organize the life of the members of his household, the Apostolic Palace, so that they joined him in a common life of prayer. He, therefore, had Litanies and various prayers recited by the members of his household towards the end of the day for the welfare of the faithful. "For he considered that the duty of a Pontiff lay chiefly in making intercession before God for the faults and necessities of his people, and that he ought, therefore, to be intimate with, as well as acceptable to, Him with Whom he was appointed to intercede. After the example, therefore, of Moses, who frequently went in and out of the tabernacle, he retired from business from time to time in order to discourse with God, that he might learn from God within what he should teach to the people without."[3]

2. *Perseverance in Prayer throughout the Day was the Early Christian Tradition*

Our Lord Himself taught us the lesson of persevering prayer: "And He spoke also a parable to them that we ought always to pray and not to faint." (Luke XVIII:1). What Christ says here of a widow seeking help in her special difficulty may be extended to our own prayers for perseverance and eternal salvation. And then St. Paul says: "Pray without ceasing" (I Thes. V:17); and again: "I will therefore that men may pray in every place, lifting up pure hands without anger and contention." (I Tim. II:8).

---

[2] Vol. I, May 1, lib. 6.

[3] See *Heroic Virtue*, I, p. 242.

None of these passages mean absolute continuity of prayer by special acts but at most prayer often repeated in the course of the day. And so they were understood in early Christianity.

Thus, Clement of Alexandria writes: "The whole life (of the perfect Christian) is a solemn festival. His sacrificial offerings[4] are prayers and hymns of praise and the holy reading to which he devotes himself before his meals, the psalms and hymns during the meal, and before he goes to bed, for at night he prays again. In this way he joins himself to the divine chorus, in unending contemplation in unceasing mindfulness. . . . Therefore, he prays in every place, but not so that it appears openly to everybody. But when taking a walk, or conversing with others, when at leisure, or during reading, or when at intellectual work, in every place he prays."[5]

Study the following passage from St. Basil and you will see that if duty robs you of your morning meditation, it does not thereby bring to an end your union with God during the whole day. "When you sit down to table pray; when you take bread: give thanks to Him Who gave it; when you strengthen the weakness of the body with wine be mindful of Him Who gave you this gift to rejoice the heart and do away with infirmities. Does the necessity of taking food pass by? Let not the memory of your kind Benefactor pass away. If you put on an undergarment, give thanks to the Giver. If you put on an outer garment, let your heart swell with the love of God, Who both winter and summer gives us suitable clothing which protects life and covers nakedness. Is the day done? Thank Him Who for the works of the day gave us the service of the sun, but fire for light in the night and to serve us in the other necessities of life. The night gives us other reasons for prayer. When you look into heaven and gaze upon the beauty of the stars, pray to the Lord of all things visible and adore God, the most excellent Creator of the universe Who made all things in Wisdom . . . . And so you will pray without ceasing, though you do not express your prayers in words, but by the whole conduct of your life, you will unite yourself to God, and so your life will become a continuous uninterrupted prayer.[6]

The way to attain to frequent prayer such as mentioned by Clement

---

[4] Clement wrote in the days of pagan sacrifices.

[5] *Stromata*, VII, vii, Migne, P.G. IX, 469.

[6] *Opera Omnia*, St. Basil, Paris, 1839, Homilia in Martyrem Julittam, 3, Vol. II, p. 50.

of Alexandria and St. Basil is not merely by resolving to think of God often and pray to Him. We must try to develop our love of God that is to live so that God will increase our charity. This means a Eucharistic life with daily Mass and Holy Communion and fidelity to mental prayer and holy reading. From such a life there may come an abiding consciousness of peace in the divine presence which is not lost during the work of the day but continues without any effort on our part to maintain it. And from this prayer rises spontaneously on every occasion. Where thy treasure is there is thy heart also. Sins and imperfections fade away and the soul attains to perfect sanctity.

3. What Manner of Prayer is Necessary for Heroic Sanctity

For those who have determined to become saints at all costs, without reference to canonization, we are interested in outlining what manner of prayer would be looked upon as pointing to heroic sanctity.

Prayer is divided into two forms: vocal and mental. Some theologians say that there is no precept of private vocal prayer, others teach that "the precept of vocal prayer was laid on every Christian who is capable of it, and that it rests on the example of Christ, and the practice of the universal Church.[7]

On the other hand there have been in the history of the Church extreme opinions on the necessity of mental prayer. The *Illuminati* in 16th century Spain taught that no one could be saved without the practice of mental prayer as taught by their masters.[8] The quietism of Miguel de Molinos (1640?-1697) tends in the same direction. Benedict XIV quotes one theologian as saying that "the note of temerity is to be affixed to the proposition that no one can be saved who does not give up some time every day to mental prayer."[9]

As a matter of fact, if you study the history of souls you will find that it is possible for one to not even know what mental prayer means and whose life has been free from mortal sin and whose biggest sin was to let the sun go down on her wrath. She said her morning and evening prayers, grace after meals, the office of the Third Order of St. Francis and some other prayers and asked: how do you make mental prayer? And yet ever conscious of the presence of Christ she made mental prayer

---

[7] Benedict XIV. Op. cit. I, pp. 238-239.

[8] *Documenta Ecclesiastica Christianae Perfectionis.* Josephus De Guibert, S. J. Rome Gregorian University. 1931, §405, 406, 407.

[9] Op. cit. I, 255.

all day long, she sang hymns to Christ as she worked and enjoyed various mystic graces.

At the same time one may practice faithfully the exercises of St. Ignatius at the regular period for mental prayer. Such a one was not conscious of ever having committed a fully deliberate venial sin. The peace of infused contemplation enters into her morning meditation— perhaps at the colloquy—and carries over into the work of the day. And God has helped her to overcome imperfections by a number of simple beautiful mystic experiences.

Taking infused contemplation to mean a quasi-perceptual awareness of the divine presence associated with a quiet glowing intense love of God along with a profound peace, which the soul knows by experience that it can never produce by its own efforts, it is a mystic grace that God gives independently of the nature of the activity of the recipient.

Saint Teresa of Avila had an ecstasy while frying fish. God may give this consciousness of His presence in various degrees during the chanting of the Divine Office. It may be accompanied with locutions reprimanding the soul for its conduct or a silent revelation of the inner mystery of God's Being, all while the recipient is chanting the psalms and attending to the actions demanded by the rubrics, or it may be dominantly only a peace that glows with the love of God. One cannot, therefore, arrange prayer on an ascending level of (1) vocal, (2) meditation, and (3) contemplation, if we mean thereby that each one of these stages represents a fixed type of prayer, one being higher than the other, and contemplation in the sense of an effort to make oneself realize the divine presence, that is active contemplation, as the highest of them all. And the reason for this is that God may give His infused contemplation in any one of these forms of prayer and lift the recipient for the time being far beyond any of them.

One could, however, say that very often and habitually these stages would represent three ascending levels. And yet one would have to acknowledge that much would depend on how one said one's vocal prayers. Thus a good nun came to St. Teresa of Avila and said: I cannot practice mental prayer. St. Teresa had her sit down and tell how she spent the period for mental prayer, and she said in saying *Paters* and *Aves*. On further inquiry it was found that in saying her Paters and Aves she lived with Christ in His Passion for hours and entered even into the prayer of Union.[10]

---

[10] *Way of Perfection* XXX. Peer's Translation II, 125-6.

Benedict XIV had considerable difficulty in finding any external signs of perfection of a candidate's prayer whether vocal or mental. He dwells on the fact that the perfection of interior prayer is something that the Church cannot know directly. He admits that an auto-biography written by the commands of superiors might be helpful. But ordinarily the perfection of vocal prayer can only be surmised by external signs such as tears; from the position and gestures of the body; from the place, time and duration of the prayer and its frequency.[11] But he points out the lack of clear definition in these signs. They form the basis of an estimate only by which those that give their suffrage must decide as well as they can "when private vocal prayer may be called excellent, perfect, and heroic."[12]

As to the necessity of mental prayer, Benedict XIV says that it cannot be termed absolutely necessary for heroic sanctity; but helps one to attain to it more easily and in greater perfection.[13]

Information on a candidate's mental prayer may be obtained from confessors and spiritual directors "likewise from the writings of the servants of God themselves, if by the command of their superiors they have committed to paper what refers to their meditations contemplations, visions and revelations."

It must be remembered that infused contemplation and mystical graces are not necessary for canonization. Sanctity is the love of God and we may grow in His love either in the dark or in the light. "Many have been enrolled in the catalogue of the Saints and the Blessed who never were contemplatives."[14]

But we might say that were it shown that a candidate did not lead a life of prayer at all, he could not qualify for beatification.

4. Opportunities for the Heroic Practice of Mental Prayer in our Busy Modern Life

Heroism often arises by the conquest of difficulties that seem in-surmountable. Parish priests whether pastors or curates will often tell you that there is no place for mental prayer in the daily duties of the modern parish. Sometimes one will say with an apparent sense of self-satisfaction: "My work is my prayer."

[11]Op. cit. I, 240.
[12]Op. cit. I, 245.
[13]Op. cit. I, 256.
[14]Op. cit., p. 270.

And yet there are priests who do find time for mental prayer in a busy city parish. A group of secular priests met together in conference and discussed the problem of finding time for mental prayer in their busy parish life. One of them wrote to me. The following is a digest of their conclusions as I remember them.

1. Give up all that does not concern us and devote ourselves to the spiritual life and our work for God.

2. This will enable us often, if not usually, to retire early enough to rise about two hours before our morning Mass, and devote ourselves, after saying Prime, to a period of prayer and holy reading.

3. When this period of prayer and holy reading must be sacrificed to our parochial duties, we will make special efforts to live with God all throughout the following day. We will slip into the church at every spare moment for a visit to the Blessed sacrament, however brief. When possible we shall say at least parts of the Divine Office on our knees before the Blessed Sacrament. Again and again throughout the day we will make acts of love and adoration to God and salute the Blessed Mother. Should it be possible to recapture the lost period of mental prayer at any time in the day, we will avail ourselves of the opportunity.[15]

Let us suppose that a busy parish priest cheerfully lived for many years according to these resolutions until his death; it seems to me that there could be no doubt about his having practiced mental prayer in an heroic degree.

Would it be necessary that such a priest should attain to infused contemplation in his periods of prayer in order to rise to true heroism in mental prayer? The answer is: No! And the reason is that infused contemplation is a special gift of God and cannot be acquired by our own efforts even by using God's ordinary illuminating and inspiring graces. And as we have pointed out, Benedict XIV says that there are many canonized saints who never were contemplatives. Furthermore, many holy souls practice prayer faithfully and never taste infused contemplation. Sanctity is measured by our love of God. Though the mystic graces, including infused contemplation, are most precious gifts and help us to love God more perfectly, it is not necessary for God to use them in order to lead us to the heights of sanctity.

In all that concerns the ideal of man and his conduct, we learn most

---

[15] *The Sister Miriam Teresa League of Mental Prayer Bulletin*, Convent Station, N.J., 1954, 9, p. 4. (October).

from a study of the character and actions of Our Lord. Let us therefore try to have a glimpse of Christ at prayer. Consider the following
passage in St. Luke: "It came to pass that as He was in a certain place
praying, one of His disciples said to Him: Lord, teach us to pray, as
John also taught his disciples." (Luke XI:1).

It was one of those occasions when Christ went apart from the
crowd and away from some village to the outlying hilly region. There,
hidden in some gully and kneeling perhaps on a dry rock, He gave
Himself up to communion with His heavenly Father and prayed for
the people He came to save. More than once the Scriptures tell us of
the Apostles seeking Him, knowing that he would be hidden some-
where in silent prayer. St. Luke here speaks of one of these occasions.
It seems that on this occasion at some little turn in the valley they came
suddenly upon Him, mute and motionless, absorbed in His communion with Him Who sent Him. The Gospels speak in several places
of something in Our Lord's conduct that gave an overwhelming
conviction that He was more than man. Thus when the chief priests
and Pharisees sent their ministers to arrest Him and bring Him before
them, they went and found Him preaching to the people. They listened.
They dared not interrupt Him. They waited till He had finished. Even
then they dared not touch Him. They returned without Him and when
the Pharisees "said to them: Why have you not brought Him?" they
said to them: "Never did man speak like this man." (John VII:46).

And when after His three hours of agony Jesus, having cried out
with a loud voice, "gave up the ghost . . ." the centurion who stood over
against Him, seeing that crying out in this manner, He had given up
the ghost, said, indeed this man was the Son of God. (Mark XV:
37-39).

When on the occasion just mentioned the disciples suddenly came
upon Christ at prayer, no one spoke. They waited silently. He did not
move. Never had they seen a man pray like this man. A divine peace
radiated from Him and entered into their very being. It was an
apostolic peace. It converted them. They wanted to pray as Christ
prayed. They waited in perfect silence till Christ rose from prayer:
"Master," they said, "Teach us to pray." It was then that Our Lord
gave to all men for all the centuries until the end of time, the words of
the *Our Father*. These words represent the prayer of Christ as the Head
of the human race. They also state what we must express or imply in
every prayer and tell us what we should pray for and strive for all the

days of our life. Our Lord still makes that self same prayer in our name as He sitteth at the right hand of God in Heaven: the Eternal Representative of the human race in the presence of the Almighty Creator of man.

Perhaps we can take occasion of this incident in the life of Christ to say something about our physical attitude in prayer. In chanting the divine office in choir it is of obligation to take a proper attitude of prayer whether standing, sitting or kneeling: no slouching, no crossing of knees. Reverence to Almighty God suggests that the same should hold of reciting the Divine Office in private. It is a solemn liturgical function and nothing should be allowed incompatible with due reverence while offering our worship in union with Christ before the throne of God in heaven. All this of course refers to a healthy man. One sick in bed says his office devoutly in bed. One ill, for instance, with heart disease, may sit instead of standing or kneeling.

As to private mental prayer one may follow the advice of St. Ignatius and take whatever attitude is conducive to devotion. But those who have a tendency to go to sleep in any comfortable position might find it wise at times to kneel or stand.

When thinking of the prayer of Christ, there is something of far more importance than our attitude in prayer and that is this. Our Lord's life of prayer was associated with self-denial. When He went into the desert to prepare for the three years of His active ministry, He not only did so to pray in solitude, but to fast for the whole forty days of his retreat and to eat nothing at all during that time. And having set that example He went forth to preach: "*Do* penance for the kingdom of heaven is at hand." (Matthew IV:17).

His whole life was a penitential life of poverty, though He could have banqueted with kings had He chosen. Instead He endured the stable of Bethlehem and the poverty of Nazareth and the nakedness of the Cross.

And then there was the spiritual sufferings of the soul: the insults and the hatred of the Pharisees. The lawyers were "lying in wait for Him and seeking to catch something from His mouth that they might accuse Him." (Luke XI:54).

Christ's last prayer on earth was His death upon the Cross. But that prayer continues into the Holy Sacrifice of the Mass. To make that prayer with Him as we should, we too must welcome as He did all the trials and sufferings of life, we must be like Him in a life of true denial of self, reasonably within the limits of our strength, and take up our cross and follow Him. All this is necessary if our prayer is to be like the prayer of Christ. Without the heroism of the Cross no prayer can be heroic.

If our sanctity is to resemble the sanctity of Christ we must not only pray but lead a life of prayer and this life of prayer must be associated with a life of penance and the patient endurance for God's sake of all the trials and sufferings of life. "If any man will come after Me let him deny himself, and take up his cross daily and follow Me." (Luke IX:23).

II. Mental Disorders and Sanctity at Its Therapeutic Level

CHAPTER XIII

Religion and Major Mental Disorders

THE PROBLEM OF religion and mental disorder is in itself one of major interest and importance. But it cannot be presented to the general reader without giving him a general conspectus of typical mental conditions known to psychiatrists, particularly those that have their roots to some extent in the stress and strain of life.

In the following chapters we shall attempt to give an understanding of the various abnormalities of mental life by drawing a picture of the individuals who suffer rather than by discussing in general terms the disorders of the mind. In this chapter we shall deal with major psychoses in what is known as the manic-depressive and schizophrenic mental disorders.

1. The Manic-Depressive Psychoses

Some years ago the author undertook a piece of research on the connection between symptoms in the major forms of mental disorder. This study was made in various mental hospitals. He went to one hospital to interview a patient suffering from what is termed the manic type of manic-depressive psychoses. He was led through various rooms, each door being locked behind him. Finally the attendant opened a door which led to a well-screened porch. He called loudly the name of the patient. In a moment a tall, powerfully built man burst into the room swinging his arms. His belt was wrapped around his clenched right hand and he looked like an ancient Greek boxer. He shouted, "Who wants to see me?" The attendant shrank back and pointed to me. He rushed at me. Then all of a sudden he took the belt from his hand, grasped my hand and said, "O! Father I am so glad to see you." He was not a Catholic, but one of those good people who respects any clergyman no matter what his denomination.

As a matter of fact, in spite of his violent manner he was not angry and intended no harm to anyone. But it is characteristic of manic patients that they do things by excess. Kraepelin gives a picture of a manic smoking: a cigar in each corner of his mouth and a pipe in each hand, looking immensely delighted with the performance.[1]

This patient looked very happy as he was talking to me. He chuckled and laughed out of a feeling of exuberance, not because of any jokes I told. He needed nothing to laugh about. His speech was rather rapid and excited. This abnormal gaiety is a characteristic symptom of manic patients. It is termed *euphoria*.

He had had a good education and was very popular in college. Popularity is likely to be a characteristic of manics before the onset of their mental disorder. He was the valedictorian of his class when he received his A.B. He then spent two more years for an M.A. He could not get ahead financially because of his mental abnormality. His moods fluctuated from depression to excitement. His depressed days were spent in bed; and on his happy days he gadded about, unable to attend to business. He was selfish and inconsiderate at home. With others he was a fine "mixer," but not intemperate. Before he entered the hospital his life was characterized by these rapid changes from excitement to depression. On an excited day in the hospital he will yell for water, and when it is brought will throw it on the floor.

Irritability, tantrums, destructiveness and euphoria are stastistically the fundamental symptoms of this disorder. Perhaps one-fourth the cases suffer from bizarre, unreasonable delusions. An attack of the manic form of manic-depressive insanity is likely to clear and to recur. But fairly often they recover completely—or have such a long normal interim that death comes before a relapse.

Let us now take a glance at the depressed type of the manic-depressive psychoses. I once followed a patient through a series of his attacks of this type of disorder, interrupted by one spell of mild manic excitement.

In a period of some years he had a series of five depressions, each lasting about a year and separated by short periods of normality or a mild manic condition. The picture that he presented in the sixth attack, which we shall now describe, was dominantly sadness associated with fear and a depression of activity that at times made it impossible for him to do anything at the place where he worked. His fear was

---

[1] I describe it from memory. Details are not exact.

that his condition might grow worse and become unbearable. His sympathetic employer allowed him to stay on, though he did little or nothing of value to the business. He was happily married and had a good income. We could find no mental cause for the onset of his depressions. The patient's own description of the development of his condition gives a clear picture of his disorder.

"The present attack began after a six month's period of normality, following a previous year of depression. I began to notice a diminution of my cheerfulness, and other slight symptoms only too well known and for which I am always on the watch. In May I was sure I was in for another attack. All the old symptoms began in mild form, such as: (a) sensitivity to heat and cold; (b) shrinking from people; (c) distaste for my work; (d) loss of energy; (e) sleeplessness and fatigue; (f) fear and uneasiness and so forth. By mid-June I was worse and continued to slip further into the slough through July, August and September. It was a bad summer and I suffered a great deal. I had no vacation and felt the heat terribly.

"My devotional attitude fell off greatly. It became a bore and then painful to go to church. I still went as often as before, but could not pray confidently and always had to force myself to go. This is mere repetition of previous experiences.

"As I regain my normal condition, I also regain my faith and confidence in God, along with all the other things in life that I anchor to. My faith and trust in God being but a human act is affected in the same manner as all my other acts.*

"God seems far away. I cannot reach Him. My prayers have no echo—no response. They fall like arrows shot against a stone wall. They have no penetration.

"I fight against this and I say: 'I believe Lord! Help thaw my unbelief!' This best expresses my attitude.

"As I improve my prayers improve; I begin to sense the Presence and to feel sure of His care. I discovered after one of my severe attacks

---

*This is not theologically correct, nor true to his own psychology. Throughout all his depressions there remains a steady blind faith that is unaffected. It is the resonance of faith that disappears because God allows it to cease. This lack of the resonance of faith is what takes place in the Dark Night. St. John of the Cross points out that similar symptoms may arise from sins and imperfections, or from weakness and lukewarmness or from some bad humor or indisposition of the body. Dark Night of the Soul I, ix, Peers Trans. I, 6. 373.

that I really loved God for the first time in my life. Not just respect or obedience or fear, but affection towards Him. I had never felt it before as much as I had desired it. So now when I recover there comes a gradual upsurge of emotion, a sense of gratitude and affection towards God. Then it becomes a pleasure to go to Mass and I am able to lift myself."[2] ·

The patient tells us how he was able to help himself by the following considerations.

"I have lately derived a bit of consolation from what to me is a new idea. I was never able to quite sincerely offer up my affliction for myself, either in expiation for past wrong-doing or as a credit for the future. This was based partly on my refusal to believe in the 'visitation of Providence' theory. In spite of the evidence of the Gospel of the sparrow's fall, I cling to the permission theory and am strongly convinced that the thing is like an attack of typhoid and due to natural causes. Somehow I have broken the laws of right living and am paying the penalty. And God permits the law to work itself out to fit His own ends. It is good for me to suffer. It is His will.

"Now to offer up this pain for myself seems a contradiction or at least it involves a sort of paradox. Maybe it is simply that I am unwilling to sacrifice myself for myself.

"But to offer it up as a sacrifice for those I hold most dear and to believe that my suffering may redound to their benefit, this is in line with my paternal instinct and this I am trying to do more or less successfully."

After fifteen months this depression passed into a hypo-manic condition.

While no psychological cause can be found for the onset of any of his periods of depression, this does not mean that the major joys and sorrows of his life have no influence on a depression once it starts. After a depression, that came on later than the one we have just described and had gone on for sixteen months, he received word that his son, a fighter pilot in France, had been shot down in his aeroplane.

"This sank me and had the following peculiar effect. It was about time for my depression to clear and those periods commenced to come when the ceiling in the mental sky lifts and one thinks that all is going to clear. But the knowledge of the boy's death kept the ceiling

---

[2] T. V. Moore, *The Driving Forces of Human Nature and their Adjustment*, New York: Grune and Stratton, 1950, p. 160. All the other data concerning this patient are taken from this source.

pretty low and my mind as it were would rise as if finally to be itself again and it would hit the ceiling: The boy is dead: there is no use getting well anyhow; and so I would sink back again. I think if it had not been for the heaviness caused by the news of the boy's death, I would have cleared sooner. But the depression hung hopelessly around me. Then one day my boy came home. He had been shot down, but had only been taken prisoner. But the joy of his return did not clear my mind; it however helped me to get better. When the lifts would come, there was no ceiling to hit. My mind could rise to any height as I thought 'my boy is not dead but living,' and after a bit I was entirely well again."

Then there was the keen sorrow of the death of his wife whom he tenderly loved. But it did not bring on a depression. His next depression came nearly a year after the death of his wife.

One purpose of this little series of pictures of mental disorders is to determine whether or not a mental disorder is essentially incompatible with sanctity. If it is, the demonstration of any mental disorder would terminate the process of beatification for any candidate for canonization. I think that this example shows that there can be mental disorders which are no more incompatible with sanctity than a physical disease like pneumonia.[3] A mental disorder patiently endured, for which we are in no way responsible, may lead to an increase of sanctity in the same way as patience in any trial.

There are many points still to be clarified on the compatibility of insanity with canonization. Père Gabriel de Ste. Marie-Madeleine speaks with special authority on this point. He asks, "Is sanctity compatible with a certain degree of psychical unbalance?"

"If the question relates to some slight mental disturbance which does not impair the personality, it is very far from being settled. From the point of view of causes of beatification, doubt concerning the existence in a servant of God of some such trouble is not a sufficient reason for immediately rejecting the cause: a very careful examination of the doubt is made. It is not actually possible to find a case in which proceedings have been continued afterwards. I could, on the other hand, point to some causes set aside, because of doubts of this nature which were not satisfactorily resolved."[4]

---

[3] On depressions in saints see pp. 209 to 213.

[4] *Conflict and Light*, Edited by Père Bruno de Jesus-Marie. New York. Sheed and Ward, 1952, p. 167.

Something depends in this matter on whether or not the mental disturbance is purely affective and the patient is free from any disturbance of judgment and reasoning. The Church must be sure that a candidate for canonization has been dominated in life by God's illuminating and inspiring grace. Any insanity that would point to conduct arising from delusions, except perhaps during a transitory delirium due to an infection, would present an obstacle to beatification.

But let us now present a patient with a depression which was not borne in a manner to increase her sanctity; the patient was seen first when she was in her middle forties:

"The course of her life had been somewhat as follows: After finishing two years of high school she went to work at 16 years of age, became a successful telephone operator, and eventually had charge of a busy office. Shortly after going to work, her baby brother was born and she took great care in planning a career for him and eventually saved her money to put him through college. When about 22 she developed an ulcer of the stomach and this plagued her intermittently ever afterwards.

"The greatest sorrow of her life, however, was the breaking of her engagement to a young man when she was about 28. From that time on she felt as if she did not have and never could have a true outlet for her affections. She naturally centered everything then on making a place for her younger brother in the world, and so she undertook to put him through college.

"When she was about 38, and her brother 21, he died and she entered into a period of low spirits and depression which lasted for some years.

"About two years after her brother's death, her mother noticed that she cried a great deal. It was at this time that her mind was haunted by thoughts of suicide. She would lie awake at night thinking about how she could put an end to her life. Though a Catholic she never opened up this matter in confession. The ulcer pains became a contributing factor by keeping her awake at night, and during her insomnia her mind was tormented by thoughts of suicide. She would picture herself dead in her coffin. And then another factor entered into the complex—the craving for sympathy. She would imagine her relatives standing by her coffin and saying: 'The poor child, how much she suffered.'

"From a child she looked for sympathy especially when sick, but seldom got it. When her stomach ulcer interfered so much with her eating that she became thin, her relatives showed some sympathy and concern. But with diet and treatment she commenced to fatten up and look well, and nobody thereafter seemed the least bit concerned. This hurt her feelings, for the ulcer pains still continued and no one seemed to care. She wished she could die and said to herself: 'If I really did die of this ulcer, then they would understand and feel sorry for me for the way I have suffered.'

"One Sunday morning after returning from Mass, her mind was all upset. She had not slept the night before and felt sad and neglected. At Mass she prayed that God would take her out of this world. After Mass her sister drove her home, but only after attending to some little duties, and so she came back late for dinner. Her older brother scolded her in an angry manner for keeping everyone late for dinner. She had expected her mother to take her part and explain matters, but she did not; her brother kept on scolding. She started to cry and went up stairs alone and no one seemed to care. She did not, however, go to her own room, but to her brother's, for she knew that her brother had a revolver there hanging in a holster. She took it out and for five or ten minutes kept saying to herself: 'I can't stand it, I can't stand it any longer.' She pointed the revolver several times at her abdomen. She told me later that she thought of the abdomen rather than the head, for she felt that if she would shoot herself through the abdomen, she would be conscious for some time before her death and she would see the family standing about her and pitying her and expressing sorrow for the cruel way in which they had treated her. Furthermore, after the deed she wanted to have a chance to go to confession before she died.

"Finally she shot herself twice in the abdomen and fell. The family heard the shots and came running to the scene. Her brother got there first and then her youngest sister. But instead of pitying, they scolded her and her sister said: 'Can't you stand anything?' After the doctor and the priest came, she expecting to die, said to her sister: 'You will be sorry you weren't kinder to me.' But instead of dying and being pitied she recovered and went to the insane asylum. After being discharged from the mental hospital, she sought psychiatric help in attempting a readjustment."[5]

---

[5] T. V. Moore, *The Driving Forces of Human Nature*. New York, Grune and Stratton, 1950, p. 155.

If the reader compares this depression with the previous one, he will see that in the former the patient's depressions came on without any immediate dependence on the trials and sorrows of life. It is an example of the manic-depressive type of psychosis. Whereas the second patient's difficulties are directly consequent upon a very difficult situation in life. Her emotions are reactions to a cognitive realization of the loss of her younger brother, and of her broken engagement. This led to a craving for sympathy which was not given, and the substitution of self-pity for the family sympathy she hoped for.

The case is an example of managing mental difficulties in a manner incompatible with sanctity. The patient endurance of the trials of life and self-sacrifice and the willing union of the sufferings of life with the Passion of Christ essential to true sanctity are all conspicuous by their absence. Unfortunately, a sense of obligation to fundamental religious obligations is not always supplemented by the ideals of sanctity. Such weakness in our love for God and our personal relations with Him is responsible for our religion failing to give the needed help in the severer trials of life.

2. Some Schizophrenic Mental Disorders
A. Paranoid Dementia Praecox.

This form of mental disorder is characterized by some or all of the following symptoms: By what is termed bizarre and rational delusions; hallucinations, sometimes in the fields of all sensations; what is known as stereotypism of speech—the apparently meaningless repetition over and over again of a word or phrase; and disorientation in space, that is, the patient does not know where he is—in a hospital or not, in his home town or not.

Let us dwell for a moment on the concept of bizarre and rational delusions. A bizarre delusion is a conviction of something that the normal mind recognizes at once as inherently impossible. Thus a patient once complained: "The man upstairs is using my brain so much that I have no time to use it myself." The normal mind sees at once that this is utterly impossible. One may think that in the abnormal mind such a delusion is a "defense reaction" against realizing its insanity. But if so, there has developed a profound disturbance of judgment. As a matter of fact special mental tests do show that most of these patients have a defect in reasoning, perception, and memory.

Comparing the emotional insanities with the dementias, cognitive defects in reasoning perception and memory are more pronounced in the dementias. "The most marked difference is in reasoning ability which is much more profoundly influenced in the dementias than in the emotional insanities."[6] The real basis for this may be a defect in the synthetic sense in virtue of which the total picture of a problem cannot be held together, so that one thing cannot be seen in relation to other things. There is not, therefore, a "spiritual" defect but an inability to make a sensory synthesis.[7]

Anyone who has attempted an analytic interpretation of dreams will see that some dreams have a profound meaning to the dreamer. But the dreamer at first does not understand their meaning. Hence conscious thought of the dreamer did not weave the fabric of his dream. By associations with one point after another in the dream its meaning is finally determined. But to weave a story with a meaning is an intellectual function not a mere series of images in the imagination. And so is the formation of a delusion. Schizophrenics, not only dream in the night, but are given to day dreaming. Their dream world sometimes becomes so interesting and appealing that they have no desire to come out of it and return to the real world of daily duty. There comes a time when they want to believe in the reality of their dream world. For the normal mind this would be impossible. But as we have just seen the dementias are associated with a defect of the synthetic sense. They can no longer see one thing in relation to another, for while they think of one thing all other things retire into the background of consciousness. Hence they cannot detect the difference between reality and the data of a dream.

Let me give an illustration of a moderately bizarre delusion. I was once making a mental examination of a patient. He was silent for a while and then he leaned over and said: "I have learned to understand what the birds are saying." I asked: "Would you mind letting me know what the birds are saying?" After a moment he replied: "They tell me that I am the only lawful heir to the throne of England." "But how can that be?" I queried. "Well, it is just this way. My name is Edmundson. Once there was a king of England by the name of Edmund. I am his son; therefore, I am the only lawful heir of the throne of England." But I objected, "There are many people now in

---

[6] T. V. Moore, The Essential Psychoses and their Fundamental Syndromes, *Studies in Psychology and Psychiatry*, 1933, 3, p. 49.

[7] See T. V. Moore, *Cognitive Psychology*, Philadelphia: Lippincott, 1939, pp. 237-270.

this world by the name of Edmundson, how is it that you out of all are the only lawful heir to the throne of England?" "You should know," he answered, "that the throne goes by inheritance to the eldest son. I am my father's eldest son; therefore, I am the only lawful heir to the throne of England."

We did not pursue the matter further. But we might suggest to the reader who is given to daydreams and vain imaginings to be careful or some day he may learn to understand what the birds are saying.

I might now very briefly present a case that will illustrate that a highly educated man is not immune to the bizarre delusions and manifold hallucinations of paranoid dementia praecox.

The patient was a man 5 feet 8 inches tall and weighed 160 pounds with an excellent muscular development. His maternal grandmother at 85 suffered from a senile psychosis with vague persecutory ideas and alternating periods of excitement and depression. When 22 he contracted a specific urethritis complicated by joint involvement and rheumatic fever a year later. He entered a profession and held a number of positions with credit and success.

The first symptoms of his mental disorder were difficulties with others in his environment to which he reacted by unreasonable worry and irritability: signs of a weakening of the personality with loss of volitional control of the emotions. Then he commenced to project on others his own attitudes towards those about him. People in his neighborhood seemed to have a peculiar attitude towards him. Restlessness, insomnia, anxiety increased and he had his first break. He thought others were spying upon him and he heard voices speaking against him. Two weeks in a sanatorium and he improved enough to be discharged.

But a week later while on a street car he "knew" that he was under close observation and the passengers were ridiculing him. He complained of tobacco smoke being blown into his room and a man on the roof peering at him.

He again went to a sanatorium. There seemed to be no great cognitive defect. He did well on general intelligence tests, but was apathetic and retarded. He improved and seemed to clear with insight.

He returned to his profession and did outstanding work. But the family situation at home became strained. He heard noises in the basement and was unable to sleep. But in spite of his ideas of reference and auditory hallucinations, he was promoted with an increase of salary.

Notwithstanding this he resigned his position to go abroad and study. His delusions of reference and auditory hallucinations continued, and soon he had to be taken to a sanatorium. He was removed to an asylum where he had to be tube fed, having refused to eat the food which he said was poisoned.

He was returned to a hospital in this country and finally committed to an asylum. He complained of a group of six, one a young lady, who were able to put him in all sorts of states of tension that caused him great discomfort. He finally became seclusive and introverted spending hours every day stretched on the benches with his face turned to the wall indulging in daydreams and fantasies. He remains well oriented in all spheres.

I have no record of intelligence tests for this admission. Perhaps the daydreaming of these patients plus emotional drives transferring blame suffice to account for many ideas of reference.

When hallucinations take on an unpleasant character they are elements in a process of transfer of blame. The patient's attainments do not rise to his hopes and expectations. This must be accounted for. The whole is something akin to the psychology of the dream. Our sensory experience does not simply vanish to appear no more, but fades rhythmically like an after image after a momentary glance at the sun. Due to the rhythmic activity of the cerebral centers, mental imagery in the normal mind is ever coming and going. But it is too weak to be noticed in waking life. But on the way to sleep in the silence of consciousness one notices visual images—mostly more or less peculiar and ever changing. The thought of the day continues into sleep and the hypnagogic hallucinations, as these images are termed, are woven into the fabric of a dream. The interpretation of the symbolism of these images gives the meaning of the dream.[8]

It is likely that in paranoid dementia praecox the rhythmic activity of the cerebral centers is pathologically accentuated. Furthermore, the patient lives as it were in a dream. The patient, dissatisfied and rebellious, weaves his accentuated imagery into a delusion of persecution and becomes perfectly certain that various persons, known and unknown, are acting on his mind. The certainity arises from the

---

[8] For details see T. V. Moore, *The Driving Forces of Human Nature*, New York, Grune and Stratton, 1950, p. 90 and *Psychol. Mon.*, 1919, *27*, pp. 387-400.

intensity of his drive to exonerate himself from blame and see in the machination of others the reason for his failure in life.

It is useless to appeal to common sense and the cold logic of reality; for he has departed from reality to live in a dream world of his own. In interviewing such patients I have occasionally heard them make a remark that betrays a hidden conviction that their notions are absurd. But I have never been able to get them to profit by that momentary flash of sound reason.

We may now ask the question is paranoid dementia praecox compatible with sanctity?

Take a glance at the biographies of the canonized saints. You will find therein men and women who sacrifice their lives and all the honor, glory, pleasures and comfort they might have enjoyed in honest peace that they might devote themselves to the service of God and man. Even the cloistered contemplative life of a Carmelite is an apostolate of prayer for the welfare of man. Witness the deep interest of St. Thérèse of Lisieux in foreign missions.

Far too common is the idea that contemplatives are introverts and are concerned only with themselves. It is a grave error. The picture of our patient "seclusive and introverted, spending hours every day stretched on the benches with his face turned towards the wall" is a picture incompatible with sanctity. Sanctity demands that forgetting self one must be wholly occupied with the service of God and the welfare of man. If a paranoid patient could be led in the early stages of his disorder to give up his dreams of the great things that are going to come to him and forget all about himself in the service of God and man, not letting his left hand know what his right hand does, his condition would not progress to dementia.

B. Catatonic Dementia Praecox.

In a mathematical factorial analysis of the symptoms of the major (essential) psychoses the following symptoms were detected as constituting signs of the group factor that underlies catatonic dementia praecox.

1. *Mutism:* That is, during their illness the patients refused to talk for long periods, measurable at least in days.

2. *Negativism:* By this was meant that the patient was unreasonably uncooperative, refusing to comply with simple, ordinary requests, was, for example, uncooperative in the examination, unwilling to give an

example of his handwriting, unwilling to sit or stand if requested, uncooperative on the halls.

3. *Refusal of food:* This symptom was considered as positive if, during the illness, the patient had gone through a spell of refusing food so as to necessitate tube feeding or severe measures to force him to eat.

4. *Stereotypism of attitudes:* This symptom was termed positive if the patient had manifested a phase or period in which he maintained himself for long periods in fixed postures, e.g. standing on one leg, maintaining a peculiar attitude and staring into space, etc.[9]

The following symptoms were associated with this syndrome: *Shut in* (more or less completely occupied with his own thoughts and having a more or less fixed and mask-like expression); *Stereotypism of actions,* an example will be given below; *Silly, apparently unmotivated giggling:* Thus "Why did you laugh?" "The devil told me to go to hell and I laughed at him"; *Destructiveness:* Tears clothes, smashes the furniture; *Loss of finer sensibilities:* dirty, unkept, soils and wets, uses vulgar language; *Irritability:* outbreaks of unreasonable anger, on the ward or even in the mental examination.

Perhaps we can introduce the description of catatonic dementia praecox by an example and explanation of *stereotypism of actions.* While examining a mental patient, I noticed that every now and then he would bend his head down and turn it right and left rubbing his neck against his collar. He was one of those patients with whom you cannot carry on a conversation, but who will occasionally respond with a laconic phrase. So I thought I would try to get an explanation of this "collar rubbing." "Why are you always bending your head and rubbing your collar?" The answer came: "If you want a drink, you nod your head, don't you?" I said: "Yes, but I don't see what that has to do with the collar rubbing." "Well," he said, "if you don't want a drink you shake your head, don't you?" "But still," I replied, "I don't understand." He answered at once with strong accentuation: "I am saying no to the spirit of fornication." Then by way of confirmation and illustration, he shook his head violently rubbing his neck against his collar.

"The patient had another peculiar mannerism. He had developed the habit of swallowing air which from time to time he would emit

---

[9] See T. V. Moore, The Essential Psychoses, *Studies in Psychology and Psychiatry,* 1933, 3, pp. 80 and 23-24.

with a tremendous belch. One day I asked him why he kept on making all these belching noises. He replied with considerable emotion in his voice: "I am belching forth the spirit of fornication."

"As a matter of fact, the patient had led a wild kind of life, drinking and going around with women while his wife was dying of tuberculosis. His mental disorder developed after her death and seems to express his remorse for the way in which he treated his wife during the last stages of her illness."[10]

His peculiar stereotypisms are very interesting and his explanation of them is a matter of great importance. Some, perhaps all, the stereotyped activities of catatonic patients have a meaning to the patients. Perhaps often, as in our present patient, the stereotypism is a symbolic but inadequate attempt to deal with the mental problem that confronts them. Our patient seems to have come to a realization of the cruelty with which he had treated his wife. He is deeply repentent, but is he truly repentent? Pyschiatrists are unnecessarily alarmed by all consciousness of guilt. But there are many things about which any man should feel guilty; and cruel treatment of a wife in her last days is one of them. He can no longer go to her and acknowledge his crime and ask her forgiveness. What can he do? The essence of genuine repentence is an honest judgment: I have done grievous wrong; and a volitional determination: I will not do wrong again. Our patient apparently knows full well that he has done wrong and his stereotypism is an oft repeated piece of evidence that he has resolved not to do wrong again.

But what is lacking? Something very important. One must go before God and say with honest sorrow: Father, I have sinned against heaven and before thee. I am not worthy to be called thy son: make me as one of thy hired servants. (Luke XV:18). One who goes to God in honest sorrow will be given to know that his sin has been forgiven and also the way in which to make reparation for the evil he has done. And here again we come to an important distinction between sanctity and some forms of insanity. In insanity one substitutes something that has no value for that which leads to eternal life. In the depressed patient we mentioned above, instead of a wholesome readjustment with a deepening of religious life and a contribution to the work of the world, there was substituted self-pity and craving for sympathy;

---

[10]T. V. Moore, The Essential Psychoses, p. 85.

and finally an attempt to force the sympathy that was not forthcoming by an attempt at suicide. In the catatonic patient, we have a
schizophrenic withdrawal from reality and stereotyped mannerisms
which symbolized but could not bring about the total reformation of
his life that was demanded.

These considerations suggest that a true appreciation of religious
values by the psychiatrist, and a moral and spiritual life which would
justify an appeal to them and help to make that appeal effective,
could often be a matter of supreme importance in the psychotherapy of
many patients.

In children psychotic disorders are not so deeprooted and malignant
as in adults. We may close this section with an account of how a
catatonic withdrawal from reality was terminated by what one might
term *environmental* therapy.

A child of four developed a catatonic condition after its mother had
entered into a psychosis and was taken to a mental hospital. Strange to
say the child was then put in an orphan asylum where all the children
were much older than itself.

When I first saw the child I found it impossible to engage it in
conversation. "At most it answered 'yes' or 'no' or echoed the last
words of your sentence (echolalia). It took peculiar attitudes, stared
into space, suddenly fell into fixed positions. *Flexibilitas cerea* was well
developed, that is, you could mold its legs and arms into any position
and there they would remain indefinitely."[11]

It seemed to me that the condition was a parataxis of recoil: but we
might well look upon it as an incipient catatonic condition in childhood. On the basis of the concept that it was a withdrawal reaction, I
appeared for the child in the juvenile court and was successful in
getting the child removed from the orphan asylum and placed in a
home where there were two or three children around its own age. In
otherwords the problem of psychotherapy was transferred from the
psychiatrist to the little children in the home.

The rapidity of the resulting cure surprised me. "The mental condition cleared up, and within a week it was laughing and playing, and
talking like other children. Traces of the *flexibilitas cerea* lasted longer,

---

[11]T. V. Moore, *Dynamic Psychology*, Philadelphia, 1924, p. 233. In the reprinting in
The Driving Forces of Human Nature. New York, 1950, p. 307, the "it" of the original
was in some way unjustifiably changed to "he". The patient was a little girl.

and could be demonstrated weeks later—though they would have passed unnoticed by one who had not seen the child when the condition was at its height.

Years later I had the child looked up and brought in to see me. She was a normal, happy, cheerful, pretty, preadolescent little girl.

Chapter XIV

Mental Disorders and the Strength of the Personality

1. "Person" and "Personality"

Webster gives as the fundamental definition of person, one that is essentially that of the Roman Philosopher Boethius (480?-524?), who lived in the days of St. Benedict. Webster defines a person as "a being characterized by conscious apprehension, rationality and a moral sense; a being possessing or forming the subject of personality; hence an individual human being."

When St. Thomas Aquinas came to define the concept of person he adopted the one given by Boethius. *A person is an individual substance of a rational nature.*[1] As St. Thomas points out that which is an individual being is found in a higher sense in rational substances that have dominion over their own acts.

The term *personality* in psychiatry has developed so that it now means what Webster defines as temperament: "the characteristic of an individual which is revealed in his proneness to certain feelings, moods, and desires, and which may depend upon the glandular and chemical characteristics of his constitution."

Mayer-Gross says that originally certain authors included the intellectual functions within the concept of personality. "On the whole, however, authors both in Europe and in America have agreed that intellectual functions were best excluded from consideration and the concept of personality restricted to the *affective and conative aspects of the individual* as a whole."[2]

To the author this restriction of the meaning of the word *personality* is a matter of regret. It would have been better to have used for this

---

[1] 1. Q. XXIX, i. Persona est rationalis naturae individua substantia. (in Lib. De Duabus Naturis at beginning of book).

[2] W. Mayer-Gross, Eliot Slater and Martin Roth. *Clinical Psychiatry*, Baltimore, Williams and Wilkins, 1956, p. 91.

concept the already current word *temperament*. This is particularly true since psychiatrists seldom if ever explain the philosophical definition of person which considers man as capable of conceiving intellectual ideals incomprehensible to sense, and capable of realizing them in himself and in his conduct by free responsible acts.

As a result, the psychotherapy of the last decades has in general treated the patient largely on the animal level. It left out of consideration, therefore, moral and spiritual ideals and the free responsible action by which only they can be attained.

2. *The Strength of the Personality*

In this connection let us first consider a phrase in Webster's definition of a person: a being possessing or forming the subject *of personality*. Since the Websterian *person* is "a being characterized by conscious apprehension, rationality, and a moral sense" its expression by an outward *personality* must involve something conscious in various ways. something intellectual and moral or immoral behavior. One should exclude neither emotions nor desires nor intellectual ideals nor moral conduct.

If you exclude the intellectual and the moral, as many or most psychiatrists have done, what is the strength of the personality? One can scarcely define it except in terms of the intensity of emotions and desires.[3]

But if you conceive of man as an intellectual being, different from animals by the presence of a power to conceive of ideals and principles then the strength of the personality becomes the power of the personality to realize high ideals and to be faithful to moral principles. The true

---

[3] Leopold Bellak has outlined a possible group of rating scale tests of "Ego" strength which, on the one hand, is to be measured by the power of the ego in resisting the overwhelming drive of the "Id" to unrestrained sexual indulgence in an alluring environment. On the other hand, the strength of the ego is measured by its success in coping with the superego: conscience demanding obedience to law. Bellak's concepts may be expressed in ordinary language by saying that sexuality is something to be enjoyed independently of marriage. It is no more a sin than eating or drinking. It is the function of the ego to resist the blind drive to excess of the Id (primitive nature) and the moral restrictions of the superego (conscience) by allowing indulgence to the unmarried only within the limits of an Aristotelian mean. But apparently nothing has been done to construct and standardize the group of tests he suggests. See his *Manic-Depressive Psychosis and Allied Conditions*, New York, Grune and Stratton, 1952, pp. 4-12.

measure of strength of personality is power to do good; for it is easy to go downhill, it takes strength to climb up the glaciers to the snow-capped peak.

3. The Church's Standard of Sanctity

As we have seen in the first part (see page 14) the Congregation of Rites at Rome has laid down a standard which a candidate for canonization must meet if the Church decides to enroll him or her in the catalogue of Saints. The standard is this:

All the theological and moral virtues with their allied virtues (that the candidate had an opportunity to practice) must be demonstrated to have existed in the candidate in a high degree of perfection, and some in an heroic degree. That means that all vices must be absent. The existence of the virtues must be demonstrated by *deeds* observed by sworn eye-witnesses or attested by authentic documents. All the evidence is presented by a *Procurator* and attacked by the *Defensor Fidei* and decisions are given by a court of judges.

There are said to be two and only two ways to canonization: (1) the way of innocence. It must be demonstrated that the candidate in an entire lifetime never committed a mortal sin. In the case of St. Thérèse of Lisieux, her Confessor Père Pichon said to her: I declare before God that you have never committed a mortal sin. Confessors familiar with the candidate's whole life are allowed to testify before the tribunal to the fact that the candidate never committed a mortal sin.

(2) The other way is the way of penance. The candidate must have lived in the practice of heroic virtue from his "conversion" unto his death without having fallen again into grievous sin. (See page 40).

This is here mentioned in order to show that such an inquiry by witnesses and the study of all the writings of a candidate in giving testimony to heroic virtue for years on end demonstrate a truly prodigious strength of the personality in the saints of God while they were on earth. But this strength of the personality is not a pure natural endowment but something purified and strengthened by divine grace.

4. Psychiatry and the Principles of Morality

The principles of right conduct are dictates of reason. Man even independently of any revelation is bound to obey them by the natural law. Unfortunately, there are psychiatrists who look upon morality as nothing more than the customs of the time and in dealing with patients who have a moral conflict they even go so far as to attempt to solve his conflict by ridding him of his concepts of morality. This practice stems from Freud.

"We are not reformers, it is true: we are merely observers, but we cannot avoid observing with critical eyes, and we have found it impossible to give our support to conventional sexual morality or to approve highly of the means by which society attempts to arrange the practical problems of sexuality in life. We can demonstrate that what the world calls its code of morals demands more sacrifices than it is worth, and that its behavior is neither dictated by honesty nor instituted with wisdom. We do not absolve our patients from listening to these criticisms; we accustom then to an unprejudiced consideration of sexual matters like all other matters; and if after they have become independent by the effect of the treatment they choose some intermediate course between unrestrained sexual license and unconditional asceticism our conscience is not burdened whatever the outcome."[4]

The Freudian attack on morality is continued in the texts of our day. Thus a recent textbook implies that the moral problems of sex arise from present social customs.

"We surround marriage with religious and civil ceremony, and by these means attempt to control heterosexual expression in keeping with our monogamous type of marriage and the social weal. By stigmatizing the extramarital sex act as sinful, and by placing it under civil control, we are able in some instances to persuade people to control these urges and to express them only in marriage. The adaptation of drives to fit the moral concepts of right and wrong according to our culture is a type of ego adaptation."[5]

Morals are not mere customs. Conscience is intellect sitting in judgment on conduct. The moral principles of marriage depend first on the concept of true friendship which is eternal; secondly, on the long period of human infancy. Even at fifteen the child is not yet ready in our modern world to fend for himself; and in fifteen years a woman might well have some seven children ranging in years down to

---

[4] Sigmund Freud, *Introductory Lectures on Psycho-Analysis*. London. Allen and Unwin, 1922, Part III, Lecture xxiii, Transference, pp. 362-363.
[5] Ewalt, Strecker and Ebaugh, *Practical Clinical Psychiatry*. New York, McGraw-Hill, 1957, p. 235.

early infancy. All this demands a stable family unit and mutual love and fidelity of husband and wife.

Opposed to this is the practice of indiscriminate sexual license under communism and its centers all over the world.

When one renounces the moral principles of marriage, he does not long maintain the sacredness of any moral principles. It was the renunciation of moral principles that made possible the atrocities that took place under the Nazi regime. And it is the renunciation of moral principles that makes Russia what it is today where at any moment without trial an honest man may be condemned to death or to slavery in Siberia.

Some psychiatrists in our country should pause to consider well whither they would lead the United States of America.

5. Weakness of the Personality and Mental Disorder

A strong personality is a wholesome personality finding its highest expression in true sanctity. A weak personality easily and often fails to rise to the ideals of human perfection. In adolescence everyone has a special type of temperament which manifests various defects. The nature of these defects predict the type of insanity that the one who has them will later develop should he become insane.

There are two main groups of the major insanities: known (1) as the manic-depressive or affective mental disorders and (2) as the schizo-phrenic.

1. The manic depressive temperament: It was early noticed that the temperament of persons who later suffered from some form of affective mental disorder showed "an increased disposition to sad and cheerful moods."[6]

Let us start out from this observation and raise the question can one who suffers from a trend to excessive sadness take himself in hand and correct his faulty disposition? We might say of such a task that it is one that should not be attempted relying solely on the natural powers of the human will. One must do his best but implore the help of God. We read thus of St. Vincent de Paul who was inclined to anger in his black moods and probably had a natural basis for an anxious depression.

"Saint Vincent had a hard struggle to acquire the equanimity

---

[6] Mayer-Gross in *Clinical Psychiatry*, Baltimore, Williams and Wilkins, 1956, citing O. Bumke, Textbook of Mental Diseases, Munich 1924.

which was so admired by all. Of a bilious temperament, he was naturally inclined to melancholy and even anger. Madame de Gondi[7] had noticed this and observed that her chaplain from time to time seemed to be more gloomy than usual; she was deeply distressed at the sight, as she was afraid he was not happy in her house. 'I turned to God' he related many years afterwards, 'and I urgently begged Him to change my dry and forbidding nature and to give me a kind and gracious spirit, and by God's grace, my watchfulness in repressing the sallies of nature has set me free in part from my black moods.' "[8]

If an emotional fault of temperament in early life is associated with mental breakdowns in later life similar in character to the defective temperament it suggests that there is not only a mere sequence but also a causal relation between the two conditions. Prevention of such mental disorders should be attempted, by the mental hygiene of the home in adolescent life. In a home like that of St. Thérèse of Lisieux a mother or an elder sister could do very efficient prevention therapy by getting children to buy souls by little acts of self-denial and so for the love of God to control their little emotional outbursts, to bob up serenely at their little tasks even when they feel gloomy and don't want to, and to be kind when they feel like saying or doing something unkind.

Let us now look at the prepsychotic temperament of what has been termed anxious depression.[9] The two outstanding symptoms in this disorder are anxiety and depression. Depression is represented by spells of the blues in early life which we have just considered. Anxiety is represented in early life by a tendency to worry and peculiar abnormal fears.

Are such worries and fears compatible with a spiritual life in deep union with God by charity and profound peace and faith in God's power to protect us from all He would not have us suffer in union with Christ dying on the Cross? "And behold a great tempest arose in the

---

[7] He served as tutor to the son of Philip Emanuel de Gondi, a French nobleman holding many high offices; and was chaplain to his household.

[8] Pierre Coste. *The Life and Works of St. Vincent de Paul.* Westminster, Md., Newman III, p. 306. Citing Louis Abelly *La vie du Vénérable Serviteur de Dieu Vincent de Paul,* Paris, 1664, 2 Vol. in quarto 4⁰. Abelly knew St. Vincent personally and was given all the documents and all the letters of St. Vincent.

[9] Close to this disorder is the retarded depression.

sea, so that the boat was covered with waves, but He was asleep. And they came to Him and awaked Him, saying: Lord, save us, we perish.

And Jesus saith to them: Why are ye fearful, O ye of little faith? Then rising up He commanded the winds and the sea: and there came a great calm." (Matthew VIII:24-26).

"Therefore I say to you, be not solicitous for your life, what you shall eat, nor for your body, what you shall put on. Is not the life more than the meat and the body more than the raiment?

"Behold the birds of the air, for they neither sow, nor do they reap nor gather into barns: and your heavenly Father feedeth them. Are not you of much more value than they?" (Matthew VI:25-26).

There is a therapeutic level to sanctity, below that of heroic sanctity, which does away with all needless anxiety. It is associated with a consciousness of living in the divine presence. This consciousness absorbs the mind to such a degree that one has no time for worry and all needless fears fade. At the same time it allows one to go about all the duties of the day and do all that is possible to prevent the misfortunes of life. I think that daily Mass and the practice of mental prayer is ordinarily necessary for sanctity to attain its therapeutic level.

But not all who go to daily Mass and practice mental prayer attain to sanctity at its therapeutic level. It would seem that to arrive at the therapeutic level of sanctity one must reach a state in the spiritual life in which, *intellectually*, one fully appreciates one's incorporation into the mystical body of Christ, dying with Him for the salvation of the world. One therefore *volitionally* accepts all the eight beatitudes; with a certain intellectual and with a certain volitional readiness prays daily to be assimilated by suffering to the Passion of Christ.

Good vocal prayer may supply for mental prayer and were daily Mass impossible, God would make good and lift the earnest soul to the therapeutic level of sanctity.

This does not mean that no saint ever suffers from a mental breakdown. We shall outline conditions in St. Francis de Sales and St. Alphonsus Liguori that closely resemble the anxious depressions we are here considering. (See pages 209-213). A good skipper can steer a boat through many a storm and he does not cease to be a good skipper if he meets a storm in which he cannot save the boat.

It is quite evident that, if sanctity commences to develop early in life and attains its therapeutic level, many souls will conquer an original trend to worry and unreasonable fears and the basis for a later anxious depression will be demolished.

2. *The shut-in type of mental disorders.*[10] The term "shut-in personality" is best verified in what was termed by a German psychiatrist, Emil Kraepelin (1856-1926): *Paranoid dementia praecox.* A Swiss psychiatrist, Eugen Bleuler (1857-1939) gave to the shut-in mental disorders a new name *schizophrenia* a word which means a splitting of the mind, the seat of the mental faculties. The verification of the meaning is found in the fact that the patient's outward behavior does not correspond with what in a normal being would be the inner emotional reaction to a situation. Thus the announcement of the death of a dear relative or an old intimate friend is met with cool indifference. Furthermore, there seems to be a breakdown of connections between the daily mental activity of these patients and the carrying on of anything useful in the home or the outside world. They are shut in. The characteristics of their prepsychotic mental temperament may be put under the following headings expressive of general trends.[11]

Shut in symptoms
The patient is slow to make friends.
He is a poor mixer.
He is anything but forward and bold.
His ordinary voice is not loud.
Nor does he behave in a loud manner when angry in the prepsychotic phase.
Delusional symptoms
He had peculiar ideas in early life.
And there appeared early a strange outlook on life.
He was visionary.
He was suspicious of others.
But with all he made progress in school.

It may now be asked what can religion have to do with the prevention of such a group of symptoms as these? And the answer is this: Religion, as a virtue, demands that a man should give to God all that

[10]Known in psychiatry as the *schizophrenic* or *dementia praecox* group.
[11]Gathered from Table 1 (in "The prepsychotic personality and the concept of mental disorder" in *Character and Personality*, 1941, 9, p. 174) by taking as significant all Yule coefficients about 0.500. The diagnoses being made on the basis of the syndromes established in *The Essential Psychoses* Studies in Psychology and Psychiatry. Catholic University of America, 1933, Vol. III, No. 3.

is due to the Creator and to his fellow men all that is their due.

We owe to God adoration and obedience to His commandments and service to our fellow men. This is summed up in the two commandments: "Thou shalt love the Lord thy God with thy whole heart, and with thy whole soul and with all thy strength and with all thy mind: And thy neighbor as thyself."

The delusional symptoms in the above list are secondary to the shut-in, "withdrawal from reality" symptoms. These lead to a life apart: to lying down and dreaming instead of going out and working. To vain imaginings of what one might become and all he could possess; that block any attempt to earn a dollar or carry out any plan in reality. Sexuality mingles with the dreaming. A drive is experienced to believe in the reality of what one only imagines and so delusions commence to make their appearance. One patient said: My dreamlife in the mental hospital is far superior to anything I could hope for in the world outside and I have no desire to be discharged.

Though the paranoid does not realize it, all this behavior is irreligious and immoral. Without at first dwelling on the ideas of God and morality a wise parent, or confessor, could in various ways interest a child in the normal activities of life. Later on he could develop a true religious spirit which is incompatible with a life of idle dreaming.

Psychiatrists in a child guidance center might well be on the outlook for the potential paranoids. Among other methods they might well make use in some way of that most powerful of all factors in the strengthening of the personality: the love of God and man.

CHAPTER XV

Character Defects and Borderline Insanity

IN RECENT TIMES a special group of personality disorders, (psycho-neuroses), has been recognized which, to a large extent, is made up of mild forms of the schizophrenic and manic-depressive psychoses.[1] We have pointed out that these types of psychosis are associated with a defect of temperament in the personality before the mental break-down.[2] We would, therefore, expect certain wide variations of normal temperamental defects to appear as personality disorders.

This renders it difficult to draw a definite line between normal variations of temperament and personality disorders and between personality disorders and a psychosis commonly termed a mental breakdown. In the same way there is no definite separation between thin men and fat men and fat men and very fat men. Someone, however, divided the stages of fatness into the enviable, the comical and the pitiable.

Let us, however, attempt to approach the problem of normal and pathological changes of mood.

1. The Emotional Zero Point

In an attempt to measure the intensity of emotional conditions we rated such affective states as irritability, excitement euphoria, sadness, tearfulness, anxiety, expecting to find that a pathological emotion would vary about a maximum frequency above zero.[3] But the expectation was not fulfilled. In all the states we measured the greatest frequency was at zero except that *euphoria*, an unreasonable

---

[1] See in *Diagnostic and Statistical Manual: Mental Disorders*, American Psychiatric Association Mental Hospital Service, 1785 Massachusetts Ave. N.W., Wash. 6, D.C. Psychoneurotic Disorders and Personality Disorders, pp. 31-35.

[2] The Prepsychotic Personality and the Concept of Mental Disorders, *Character and Personality*, 1941, 9, 169-187.

[3] *The Essential Psychoses and Their Fundamental Syndromes*. Studies in Psychology and Psychiatry. 1933, III, No. 3 Catholic Univ. America, Washington, D.C.

unmotivated gaiety, has a maximum frequency a little above zero, at what we might regard, for this emotional manifestation, as the normal cheerful state of the human mind.

You may symbolize the human emotions by a circular disk with well-marked diameters passing through it at various angles. This disk is pivoted at its center. It fluctuates like a seesaw along the lines of the various diameters with a movement which is somewhat complex when various emotions are involved. No normal man has his emotions fixed in all directions. Normal life is a continual emotional fluctuation tilted upward toward a gentle gaiety.

A pathological emotional disorder is an overtilting in one direction to such an extent that the plane does not tilt back again. There is something to be said for the concept that shock therapy in the mental disorders involves a violent physiological jar to the emotional plane which gives it a chance to resume its normal fluctuations.

2. *Normal Emotional Fluctuations*

To what extent can my emotional plane tilt without my suffering from a "personality disorder?" How far must it tilt before I enter into a psychosis, or as it is said, have a nervous breakdown?

We have some data on the "diameter" on which, at its high end, one is elated, happy, cheerful and at the low end, sad, apprehensive, worried. Normal men have definite fluctuations of mood. In the "highs" a worker accomplishes more. His daily job seems to require no effort. He is cheerful, sometimes overtalkative and takes part in various outside activities. In the "lows" he is more or less peevish, disgusted, sad. The daily job becomes a drag. He feels more like staying home at night rather than going out to some amusement. In general the sleep of working men is not disturbed during their lows.

All this may be termed a normal manic-depressive cycle. The strange thing is that its duration is a characteristic of the individual. In Hersey's study from which these data are derived the duration of the cycle ranged from 3·00 to 9·25 weeks.[4] The author found one normal man in whom there was a weekly depression. It started toward the

---

[4] Rexford Brammer Hersey, *Workers' Emotions in Shop and Home*, Philadelphia. Univ. Penn. Press, 1932, and *Seele und Gefühl des Arbeiters*, Leipzig, Konkordia-Verlag, 1935. Hersey worked with workers in the United States and in Germany. He studied only 5 normal healthy women and found in them a manic-depressive cycle independent of menstrual period.

end of the day when everything commenced to be hopeless. But on the next morning it was all gone. In another the waves of depression dropped lower and lower as the house got colder while the winter advanced, but rose rapidly with the coming of spring. In a period of severe storm and stress "incidents" cloud the normal rhythm.

A man holding an important position once consulted the author about his periodic depressions. We made a study of his manic-depressive cycle. It had a duration of 26 to 28 days. But the important thing was that the depression lasted only 2 to 3 days. During it he was convinced that he was incapable of carrying out the duties of his position and felt difficulty in resisting a strong impulse to resign. Learning that he only had to wait a day or two enabled him to look forward with hope to the moment of clearing; and so it became easier to carry on knowing that he would not have to wait long for relief.[5]

3. The Entire Range of Emotional Fluctuations

We have just given an account of some of the experimental work on normal fluctuations of mood. Some years ago the author attempted to divide the reactions to the difficulties of life, which could not well be regarded as psychoneuroses, into two classes the *psychotaxes* and the *parataxes*.[6] The psychotaxes are normal tendencies to adjust oneself to the difficulties of life, whereas the parataxes go beyond normal limits towards the *psychoneuroses*. Still further beyond the limits of the normal are the extreme reactions that give us the picture of the major insanities: the *psychoses*.

When we speak of reactions or tendencies to adjust oneself to the difficulties of life we must realize that consciousness plays a part. Malingering or pure pretense is not a parataxis but a voluntary

---

[5] Winifred Bent Johnson studied "Euphoric and Depressed Moods in Normal Subjects" (*Character and Personality* 1937-38, *6*, 79-98; 188-202). The periods of her observations were not long enough to check fully Hersey's findings of "rhythms" characteristic of individuals, but many of her subjects (30 college women) had a "rhythm" of 15 days. She noted that in her normal subjects the *euphoric phase is much larger than the depressed*. Furthermore the average mood of all subjects is a mild euphoria (graph p. 83). In depressed phases the feeling of "physical energy" is reduced along with loss of confidence in one's own powers. Studies sometimes fail to find the "Hersey rhythm" because they employ too few subjects and do not follow them for a long enough period. e.g. Don W. Dysinger, The Fluctuations of Mood, *Psychol. Record*, 1938, 2, 115-123.

[6] See T. V. Moore, *Dynamic Psychology*, Philadelphia, Lippincott, 1924, pp. 182, ff and *The Driving Forces of Human Nature*, Grune and Stratton, New York, 1950, 268 ff.

adjustment with full conscious insight. From total lack of insight we
have parataxes with various degrees of conscious insight on up to total
lack of insight into the fact that one's behaviour is to some extent one's
own personal responsibility.

We may now clarify the problem by trying to define what is meant
by a *psychoneurosis*. "Psychoneurotic reactions are the commonest
modes of faulty responses to the stresses of life, and especially to those
inner tensions that come about from confused and unsatisfactory
relationships to other people . . . The pathology of psychoneurotic
reactions, in other words, is essentially a pathology of interpersonal
relations."[7]

The symptoms of a psychoneurosis may be bodily or mental or both.
The bodily symptoms may consist in areas of loss of sensation, or
hypersensitiveness, pains, headaches, palpitations of the heart, etc. or
paralyses, tics, convulsive movements. The mental symptoms may
consist in such things as unreasonable fears or movements which the
patient feels compelled to repeat again and again.

There is one characteristic which is often mentioned in case histories
of these patients: the patient becomes incapable of carrying on his
daily duties. Incapacitation may serve as a sign to distinguish between
a parataxis and a psychoneurosis.

"A psychoneurotic patient may be disconcerted by a morbid fear of
travelling in a train, or a bus, or he may be unable to go more than
a few yards from his own door, but he does not have the faintest notion
why; yet this fear may be so impelling that the attempt to walk a few
yards in the open may prove utterly beyond him."[8]

If a fear troubles one but does not incapacitate him for duty, he
may be regarded as suffering from a parataxis not from a psychoneurosis. Normal men have one or more parataxes, but normal men
do not suffer from a psychoneurosis.

The psychoneurotic symptoms are not related to any disorder or
injury to the nervous system. They seem utterly unreasonable to the
patient and to others. But when analyzed by the psychiatrist, their
mental roots often become clear. The treatment of the psychoneuroses
consists in their analysis. When the true cause is understood by the
patient the morbid symptoms usually promptly disappear. (See below

---

[7] *A Textbook of Psychiatry* by Sir David Henderson and the late R. D. Gillespie and
   Ivor R. C. Batchelor, Oxford Univ. Press 8th Ed. p. 151-152.
[8] Henderson and Gillespie, op. cit. p. 152.

page 130 for a discussion of the concept that a psychoneurosis does not come and go in spells but persists until death unless cured completely). Was St. Thérèse incapacitated by her scruples or only troubled? There is a passage in the English translation which suggests that she was incapacitated. "I must now go back to the subject of my scruples. They made me so ill that I was obliged to leave school when I was thirteen."[9] But the manuscript copy does not refer the necessity for leaving school to scruples but to her separation from Céline. The words of St. Thérèse herself are as follows: "At the end of the year, Céline, having finished her studies, returned home and the poor Thérèse obliged to go back alone soon became sick: the sole charm which kept her at boarding school was to live with her inseparable Céline. Without her, 'her little daughter' could not remain there. I therefore left the abbey at 13 years of age and continued my education by taking several lessons a week at the home of Madame Papineau."[10]

While at the Abbaye des Benedictines, Thérèse "was obedient, showing a minute fidelity to the smallest detail of the rules."[11] She adjusted to school life. When she left to go to Madame Papineau she again adjusted. When she entered Carmel she adjusted to all even to some who were hard to please. Happiness in interpersonal relations was a characteristic trait of St. Thérèse. We would not expect, therefore that she could be diagnosed as suffering from a psychoneurosis whose pathology is essentially a pathology of interpersonal relations.[12]

Like many children she manifested in childhood what is well known as homesickness. Thérèse does not tell us just how she was sick. But it is well known that "unhappiness" can provoke a number of gastrointestinal reactions.[13] And pain from such conditions may be referred to the region affected or to an area widely separated from that region.[14] Return home cured the "sickness." One cannot look upon a transient

---

[9] Soeur Thérèse of Lisieux Trans. by T. N. Taylor, New York, Kenedy 1924, p. 66.
[10] Manuscript 40 left.
[11] Frances Parkinson Keyes, *Thérèsè Saint of the Little Way.* New York, Julian Messner, 1950 quoting the unpublished "souvenirs" of one who knew her at the Abbaye. P. 77.
[12] Henderson and Gillespie, *A Textbook of Psychiatry,* p. 152.
[13] For a study with many references to the literature see Walter C. Alvarez, "Ways in which emotion can affect the digestive tract." *J. Am. Med. Ass.* 1929, *92*, 1231-1237.
[14] Ch. H. Best and Norman B. Taylor. *The Physiological Basis of Medical Practice.* Baltimore, Williams and Wilkins, 1955, p. 597 ff.

attack of homesickness in a child as a psychoneurosis. This is particularly true in one who left her home at about fifteen years and lived a normal life in a Carmelite convent until her death some ten years later.

4. Over the Borderline into a Psychosis

The difference between the psychoneuroses and the major insanities (psychoses) has been thus described: "A psychosis involves a change in the whole personality of the subject in whom it appears, while in the psychoneuroses it is only a part of the personality that is affected. With the development of a psychoneurosis there is often no outward change of personality of any kind. As Adolf Meyer puts it: "A psychoneurosis is a part reaction, while a psychosis is a total one."[15] One easily sees this in the schizophrenic psychoses with their peculiar behavior, bizarre delusions and hallucinations. And also in the wild excitements and homicidal trends of the manics. But it is also evident in the deeper depressions. Consider the following characteristic description of a profound depression: "Palid, immovable the melancholic bears on his face the marks of his anguish, . . . the head bent forward, the body is limp, drooping, bent and as it were bowed low under its weight. Seated in an arm chair or a couch or in bed, the patient makes almost no kind of a gesture and never comes out of his semimutism except to moan, sigh, groan. It seems as if all the instincts of life were abolished. He even refuses to eat and has to be tube fed."[16]

But there is another type of the depressive psychoses in which the patient is not depressed but intensively active. They pace the floor, wring their hands, pull at their hair. They may constantly cry about having committed the unpardonable sin, or being the cause of all the evil in the world. Here again there seems to be a change in the whole personality.

The problem of distinguishing between a psychoneurosis and a manic-depressive condition is complicated. Kraines has pointed out that a psychoneurosis is a chronic character defect due, as the name suggests, to psychic rather than organic causes. There is no such thing as repeated passing attacks of a psychoneurotic condition. Because it is due to mental causes it can be cured only by psychotherapy. Shock

---

[15] Sir David Henderson, R. D. Gillespie and Ivor C. Batchelor, *A Textbook of Psychiatry*, Oxford Univ. Press, London, 8th Ed. 1956, p. 156.

[16] Jean Delay. *Les Désrèglements de l'humeur*. Paris Presses Universitaires de France, 1946, pp. 9-10.

treatments do not affect it. It is a disease entity in its own right; and a manic depressive disorder is another specific disorder of the mind. Hence a psychoneurosis may pre-exist, coexist or postexist an attack of manic-depressive disorder.[17]

When we come to the duration of a psychoneurosis it is likely to last from its onset to death unless it is successfully treated by psychotherapy. A manic-depressive disorder on the other hand comes and goes independently of great sorrows or important successes. (See case history, page 101ff).

In an investigation of 556 cases it was found that "the usual psychoneurotic had great difficulty giving the exact onset of his illness or even separating it from the course of his life. A manic-depressive generally has little difficulty separating the symptoms of his illness from the natural course of his life."[18]

As to duration, a manic-depressive condition has been found to last for periods of an hour or two on up to many years. One is likely to question the right to call a depression lasting only an hour an attack of manic-depressive insanity, nor could one do so except in patients followed for years. But it has been found that brief attacks of only an hour or a week lengthen as the patient grows older, and give the characteristic picture of a true depression repeated and repeated again for many years. This makes one renounce any effort to distinguish between normal fluctuations of mood and manic-depressive insanity by the length of the attack. The coming and going of attacks of itself excludes the psychoneuroses.

An important sign of a major psychosis is a strong positive drive to commit suicide. It is one thing to have ideas of suicide come into the mind. It is another to experience a drive to kill oneself. I remember a young girl who was brought to me many years ago. She was sad, yet not deeply depressed, but determined to kill herself. She talked coldly about the *fact* that she was going to kill herself. I asked for an agreement that as long as she was coming to me her suicide would be postponed and that she would let me know if she intended to break the agreement. One day she came in and said: The agreement is off. I was unable to change her mind. So I notified her relatives. She went willingly to a mental hospital, stayed there for about a year and was

---

[17]Samuel Henry Kraines, *Mental Depressions and Their Treatment.* New York, MacMillan, 1957, p. 298.

[18]Sidney Taracho Tarachow et alii, New York, *Hillside Hospital* Journal, 1956, 5, p. 54.

discharged. She went to work. But at her first vacation went to
Niagara Falls and took a room in a hotel. The next morning at breakfast she chatted normally with the waitress and went in a cab to the
Falls. A policeman saw her. She had climbed a fence and stood at the
edge of the rapids. He motioned to her to come back, but she paid no
attention. He started to climb over the fence to get her. She waved her
hand to him, jumped into the rapids and was gone.

It is a serious responsibility to decide whether ideas of suicide are
empty anxieties or positive drives of a dangerous character. There are
ideas of suicide and also of homicide that are unreasonable fears and
not drives. A mother or a nurse will be tormented by a fear of killing
the children, but the fear is sometimes a sign that they will never kill
the children.

In what seems to be schizophrenic borderline conditions, delusions
may be evidence that there is something more present than a mere
abnormality of the personality. One man, apparently perfectly normal,
developed the delusion that he was being followed by persons who had
some kind of evil intent towards him. He therefore carried a revolver.
One night he suddenly turned around, shot and killed a man innocently
walking behind him. He was sent to a hospital for the criminally
insane. He was highly educated and his brother supplied him with all
the books he wanted. So he started making an investigation of the use
of English words from their first appearance to the present day,
writing out quotations to exemplify their use. It was the time when Sir
James Murray was editing the Oxford English Dictionary. He sent
his work to the editor. Sir James thanked him for his contributions and
sent him checks as they came in. He grew interested and in one letter
the check was accompanied by an invitation to have tea with him and
Lady Murray in London. He replied that circumstances over which
he had no control made impossible the acceptance of his kind invitation. Sir James wrote back delicately offering to defray his expenses
and our patient again excused himself by the circumstances over
which he had no control. One day, Sir James being in the city, took
a cab to our patient's address and it drew up at the hospital for the
criminal insane.

Our patient's brother, living in the United States, arranged to have
him transferred to a hospital in this country. In some way the patient
heard of me and arranged for a visit. We had a delightful conversation
and he appeared mentally normal in every way and the very type of

a perfect English gentleman. As he was going he expressed a desire to make some remuneration and I naturally replied that our pleasant conversation was sufficient remuneration. But he said: Would you not like to know how to close a door, without using lock and key of any kind, so that it can't be opened? I expressed the idea that it would give me great joy to have such valuable information. He took from his overcoat pocket a bag of small screws and pressed one in the crack between the door and the doorjamb. "Now", he said, "no one can open it till I take out the screw." "Shall I try?" "Certainly," he said, "but it is impossible." I took hold of the knob, opened the door and the screw fell on the floor. "O!" he said with a strong English accent, "you did open it, didn't you?" We chatted for a few moments and as he parted he bowed respectfully, handed me the bag of screws which I graciously received and said to me: "I hereby leave with you the means of carrying out the great secret."

One might take it as a general principle that anyone who harbors a delusion which is patently impossible is suffering from a psychosis no matter what the apparent normality of his personality. When, however, the patient's delusions do not bring him into conflict with his surroundings, such psychotic individuals often live harmless and even useful lives outside of an institution. I might mention a man famous in the history of philosophy for a special piece of research, who was invited to give a series of lectures at one of our great universities. He visited me and on parting asked if I would like to have the secret of all wisdom. I said: most certainly. He got a glass of water, sat tailor fashion on the floor, started to make quick violent passes with one hand over the glass of water, and held his nose tightly closed with the other hand while he gulped down the glass of water. He then looked up and said solemnly: "Do that and you will have the secret of all wisdom."

5. Personality Disorders and the Mental Troubles of Persons

It is characteristic of Freudian psychotherapy to minimize the mental stress of the present moment and pay little attention to individual types of character while the whole object of the analytical procedure is to unearth a traumatic sexual episode in childhood. But if the personality of an individual can be weak by reason of heredity, the stress and strain of life or inadequate training, can one hope to treat *all* mental disorders by confining the therapeutic technique to the search for sexual traumata in early childhood? And if a patient is not helped by Freudian analytic technique is it good psychiatry to dismiss him as incurable?

If it has been established as even solidly probable that there is a group of mental disorders the origin of which is rooted in the inadequacy of the personality, should not the study of a mental patient involve an investigation of the nature and extent of the defects of his personality? And that having been done, and various personality defects noted, should not an important element in the therapeutic procedure be the adoption of measures to reorganize and strengthen the personality?

We shall point out below the importance of religious factors in psychotherapy. (pp. 136ff and 144.).

We might now ask the question: Is the religious factor in psychotherapy limited only to those who have already attained a high level of sanctity? The answer is that sanctity at the therapeutic level acts efficiently by its very existence; but any human being, no matter how low he is in the depths of immorality, if he turns to God with all his heart and asks for help, will surely get it.

6. Psychotherapy and miracles

We must here make a distinction between two kinds of help that God gives to those in need.

1. That which is miraculous and beyond all the laws of nature and the working of God's ordinary grace.

2. That which is not beyond the laws of nature and within the sphere of action of God's ordinary grace.

The scientific world in general does not recognize the existence of miracles, but in this it is unreasonable. Only recently a woman told me of her young child who had a large palpable mass in the abdomen. The laboratory technician came to make a blood test. Going back to the laboratory he found the blood normal. Thinking that there must be some error he returned and made another test. This was also normal. He notified the specialist who examined the child. There was no palpable mass, and the child was playing around like any normal infant. The family had been making a novena for the child's recovery.[19]

---

[19]Anyone who reads *The Miracle of Lourdes* by Ruth E. Cranston (a non-Catholic) New York, McGraw-Hill, 1955 (with the testimony of Dr. S. Oberlin that the accounts of the cases in the book are in accordance with the records and findings of the Medical Bureau and Medical Commission of Lourdes) will be unable to reasonably deny that miracles are facts. The writer visited personally many who had been cured after having studied the official documents.

But when speaking here of religious factors in psychotherapy we have no intention of bringing in the miraculous. Nor do we expect religious psychotherapy to be applied to the treatment of organic conditions such as fractures and cancers and infectious diseases. But it has its place among psychotherapeutic procedures—especially in mental conditions when all other types of psychotherapy have failed.

7. Psychotherapy Without Reorganization of the Personality

Let us take a case studied and presented by the staff of the psychiatric service of the Massachusetts General Hospital, Boston.[20] Some of those at the conference regarded the case as an example of *psychoneurosis anxiety*. Thus it might be brought under the caption of the borderline psychoses we are here considering as personality disorders.

The presenting symptom was a tremor of the hands which gave rise to intense unreasonable anxiety. The condition developed when the patient was given a promotion, moved out of his shop and made general inspector of various shops operated by the company.

This intensified a chronic defect of temperament: he had always found it difficult to meet and converse with strangers. He then noticed the trembling of his hands. He had to dine with others and the trembling made eating and drinking very difficult. With the trembling there came on sweating, increased tension, palpitation, easy fatigability and insomnia. He often missed meals rather than eat with others. He lost weight and quit work. After a month he went back to his old job as machinist. But his symptoms instead of being alleviated were intensified.

He became disgusted with himself and started drinking heavily. He attempted suicide by swallowing rat poison. This had little physical effect on him, but added remorse of conscience to his mental troubles.

A physician diagnosed his condition as due to thyroid trouble. But iodine therapy had no effect.

Physical examination suggested psychotherapy.

The first stage in the psychotherapy was merely to point out to the patient the types of situation that "provoked his anxiety symptoms." He accepted this but did not see how it would help him. He feared he would never get better.[21]

---

[20]*Case Histories in Psychosomatic Medicine*, Edited by Henry H. W. Miles et al. New York, Norton, 1952, pp. 189-202.

[21]Op. cit. p. 194.

Later psychotherapy seems to have been directed at discovering a castration complex[22] "Using examples from the patient's productions it was possible to point out to him how his fears and feelings of inadequacy were associated with feelings of guilt and self-depreciation because of his belief that he was a weakling and not a real man."[23] This was an attempt to trace all his present anxieties to castration threats by his parents and a surgical operation for hernia in childhood. Such specific threats were not found but only the general threats of some kind of punishment.

The final result was no improvement and slipping back to his old solution of heavy drinking.

"At the present time the patient seems well on the way to solving his problems by becoming an alcoholic like his father."[24]

The analysis, treatment and final outcome of treatment in this case raises the question: What percentage of cases of anxiety arising or being increased in later years are due to castration threats by parents in childhood? There is a tendency among analysts to speak of a castration complex existing whenever a child has been threatened with any kind of punishment. With this interpretation most human beings suffer from a castration complex.

The patient had a long standing character defect: difficulty in meeting and conversing with strangers.

The weakness of his personality was also evidenced by a resort to heavy drinking instead of confronting his problem and carrying on to the best of his ability. Any person who is morally inadequate has a character defect. A bridge, too weak for the traffic it has to support, can be strengthened.

But the fashion in various quarters of present day psychiatry is to neglect the bridge and the strain of traffic and look for conflicts among the builders, while the bridge was being erected, which has nothing to do with the materials employed in its construction, or the strain of traffic.

8. Reorganization of the Personality

The reader is probably asking: how can the psychiatrist reorganize the personality of the patient?

[22]Op. cit. p. 198 ff and 201.
[23]P. 199.
[24]P. 200.

Let us first look at what constitutes a normal personality or character. A normal personality is a personality well adjusted:

(a) in his own interior life with stable control of his emotions; and with a worthwhile ideal in life towards which he is honestly and effectively striving, with conduct governed by sound moral principles.

(b) who is well-adjusted in his family life, loving all and free from antagonisms or hatred towards anyone.

(c) and who is in like manner well-adjusted where he works and to the society in which he moves.

(d) and finally well-adjusted as a rational creature should be towards God, the Creator.

The following active causes of mal-adjustment may be mentioned:

1. The lack of anything like a worthwhile ideal in life.

2. The lack of sound moral principles.

3. A spirit of rebellion to home and society often due to unwise management of the child by parents.

4. No knowledge or very deficient knowledge of God and religion.

5. To these may be added traumatic shocks in the past giving rise to special disability of conduct.

6. Organic defects of emotional control. These render difficult but do not make impossible the reorganization of the personality.

7. Excessive mental strain due to major calamities in life.

Sometimes religious therapy alone can help in these situations. But when the patient has no adequate religious background it may be humanly impossible to get him to cooperate in religious psychotherapy.

Modern analytic psychiatry, as in the case just presented, is likely to give excessive attention to number 5 and center all in tracing symptoms back to traumatic shocks in the past. Sometimes this will be misplaced effort and the patient will not be helped.

Often, especially in adolescent problems the key to the situation is the crystallizing of a worthwhile ideal in life and the establishing in the mind of sound moral principles, culminating in the development of the relation that a human being should have to God, his Creator. One must start at the bottom with the moral principles and the ideals of life.

Something can be done here in a series of interviews with the patient. But one must carefully avoid giving the impression that one is trying to preach his own principles to the patient. One is very much helped here by a little library in his office of some two to three hundred books labeled for reading level. They must be very interesting and

naturally free from anything immoral.[25] It is best to select a book with
a problem akin to that of the patient. But it is not necessary. The
patient reads his problem into or out of the book, just as a trivial
incident of the day is the starting point of the dream of the night.
Much depends on the skill with which the therapist discusses the book
with the patient. The patient will discover what he regards as "his
own" moral principles from his reading. The therapist by questioning
may help him to formulate them.[26]

Religious psychotherapy as an adjunct to other methods is difficult
or impossible in patients without adequate religious development. Few
psychiatrists can utilize it, but at times no other method will give any
help. For this reason when the staff of a hospital meets to consult about
a patient, a *specially trained* chaplain of the hospital might well sit
in consultation and should often take part in the therapy. Already the
Department of Psychology and Psychiatry at the Catholic University of
America at Washington is offering a program of courses leading to an
M.A. or Ph.D. for priests who are destined by their Bishops to be
hospital chaplains.

Many psychiatrists of the present day still think that all religion is
an evil. But the old order changeth and giveth place to new. That
transformation is taking place in psychiatry at the present day.[27]

---

[25]Clara Kircher, *Character Formation Through Books, A Bibliography*. Washington, D.C.
Catholic University of America Press, 1944.

[26]For an illustration of the technique of reorganizing the personality see T. V. Moore
The Driving Forces of Human Nature. New York, Grune and Stratton, 1950, pp. 388-
396.

[27]*Proceedings of the Fourth Annual Psychiatric Institute*. Held September 19, 1956 at the
New Jersey Neuropsychiatric Institute. Princeton, N.J.

CHAPTER XVI

Shock and Selfishness in Personality Disorders

A SUDDEN EMOTIONAL shock, let us say, from seeing a child killed may result in a major mental disorder. It is not surprising, therefore, if we find that sudden sorrows, personal calamities or the imminent danger of death may bring on transient or permanent minor disorders of the personality.

Psychiatrists had long been familiar with these facts at the outbreak of the First World War. There were two schools of interpretation: One, the brain physiologists to whom all mental disease meant brain disease. But Freud was already showing by his psychoanalysis that some mental disorders had their origin in mental experiences.

Early in the First World War the public heard much of peculiar disturbances caused in apparently uninjured men by shells that exploded close to where they were stationed. They became blind, but their eyes remained intact. They were paralyzed without any injury to muscles or nerves. They developed bizarre convulsive movements of arms and legs that made it impossible for them to stand at their posts and handle a rifle. They were made deaf but there was no injury to the tympanic membrane or anything else in the ear.

The "brain physiologists" found a ready explanation of such conditions in a concussion experience which shook up the molecules in the brain and perhaps also caused tiny hemorrhages in regions concerned with the symptoms manifested by the patients. But neither in war psychoses nor in the cases of shell shock (termed war neuroses) could there be found, in general, any actual injuries to the brain, let alone just such injuries as might be expected to account for the symptoms.

As experience developed it was found that some peculiar symptoms of shell shock manifested themselves on the patient's being drafted, or ordered to France, or going into the trenches and perhaps stumbling over the dead body of a soldier, before any shell exploded to cause the patient to suffer from shell shock.

139

As the war neuroses were studied it became apparent that they were often what was termed defense reactions rendering duty in danger of death impossible. Evasions of duty are self-seeking reactions rooted in human selfishness.

There are, however, emotional shock reactions that are the result of a sudden profound emotional reaction in which selfishness does not play a part. We shall commence our study with one of these and lead on to the unmanly evasion of the war neuroses.

1. Emotional Shock Reaction

Let us start with an illustration of a shock reaction.

A young married woman of 26 came with the following major complaints:

1. I have been scared to death about something all my life and I don't know what it is.

2. I have been bothered by frequent headaches for nearly two years.

The following attempts at psychotherapy were made:

1. Taking the personal history of the patient as far as emotional events could be recalled without any analysis. This threw no light on her present problem: "scared to death about an unknown something."

2. An attempt at analysis by free association. This brought out the existence of much tension in her home before her marriage. There was constant quarreling between her father and mother; and also the way in which she blocked her father's attempts to give her a higher education, by spending her time in dancing and going to the movies.

3. A technique advocated by Adolf Meyer: have the patient write out a detailed account of the emotional difficulties of past life and discuss them with the psychiatrist. It is rather interesting to note that discussing this patient's emotional history led to the unearthing of a buried emotional shock experience. Its recall led to an "abreaction" that was followed by an immediate clearing of the fear about an unknown something that had "scared her all her life."[1]

In her general history she mentioned that she was an only child. When she was about 8, her parents took into the house three of her

---

[1] See on this patient T. V. Moore, *Nature and Treatment of Mental Disorders*, New York, Grune and Stratton, 2nd Ed., 1951, p. 104 ff.

boy cousins who had been left orphans when about 11, 7½, and 4 years of age. "They had all been very ill with typhoid, and the baby was quite helpless when he came to us. For as long as he was with us, he was the center of my world."

"In the interview which took place when she brought in her emotional history, she told how she was looking on when her little cousin was burned so severely that he died shortly after. He and some boys had found a can of gasoline and were pouring it on the ground and setting fire to it with matches. While her little cousin was holding the can, one of the boys held a match over the opening. An explosion followed and the little fellow was wrapped in a sheet of flame. Both his hands were almost burned off."

After a few associative recollections she came to an incident which she had tried to keep out of her mind for fourteen years.

"When my younger cousin, the boy who died so horribly, was about 8 years of age and I was 12, he and the older boys and myself were in the kitchen one night. I have forgotten whether we were doing the dishes or just what we were doing, but I do remember that there were dishes and kitchen utensils of all kinds near me. The older boys had been teasing me about something, I have forgotten what it was now, but it seems that I had taken quite all I could stand. I am not very clear about what followed immediately afterwards, but the next thing I knew Frank (the little boy who was later burned to death) had one of the heavy two pronged kitchen forks stuck in his wrist. I know I did not mean to hurt him. I don't even remember picking it up, but I must have done so. It seems as I look back now as though all this unreasoning fear dates from that night. I have an ungovernable temper, and it takes all the strength I have to keep it under any kind of control. The only thing I have found of help is to leave any argument before it gets to the proportions of a fight, and go out and walk until I have calmed down. I have never thrown anything from that day to this, but still I believe I am afraid of what might happen."

When the patient came to this point in the interview she manifested what Freudians would term an *abreaction:* giving full vent to a buried emotion when the incident that originally caused it is brought to consciousness and talked over freely. The patient became pale, an expression of anxiety came over her face and her voice trembled. She said: "This is the something I have been scared to death about all my life and now I know what it is." There had been a deep sense of guilt about having pierced her little cousin's wrists with the two pronged fork. And then she had seen him wrapped in flames and when she got to him his two hands were almost burnt off.

We continued to talk about her difficulty and she said that she now feared that she might kill someone in her anger.

I then attempted to help her to a complete cure by considerations of reason and common sense. I explained that the anxiety about killing someone was not based on reason and common sense, but on an anxiety rooted in the unfortunate experience she had just unearthed after years of repression. I dwelt on the fact that there comes a period in the maturation of the personality in which normal individuals no longer throw things or strike or carry on like children in their anger. She was no longer a child and had every reason to expect that she would not again behave like a child when provoked to anger.

Whatever criticisms may be made of our technique of therapy, it was completely successful. It was remarkable to see how in the next interview the patient seemed a very different type of individual: so cheerful and happy that one would never have believed that for fourteen years she had suffered chronic anxiety about a hidden something and did not know what it was. She returned for two more visits, separated by a period of some weeks, and remained a perfectly normal cheerful individual. As she expressed it, "There has not been a bit of trouble since that analysis."

2. Fears of Special Objects

In the patient just presented there was a gnawing vague anxiety of something she knew not what. Such a condition is sometimes termed simply an *anxiety reaction*. On the other hand patients have a fear of some kind of particular object: dogs, snakes, mice, spiders, bugs, high places, going round a curve and host of other *phobias,* the intensity of the fear being out of all proportion to the object. Very often the person who has such a fear recalls the incident in which it originated. John Edward Wallace Wallin made a study of some hundreds of these phobias. He concluded that a phobia may develop on the basis of any intense emotional experience. Thus for instance he reports the following case:

"My first conscious fear was of dogs. At the age of 5, I saw my dearest playmate bitten and lacerated by a huge mad dog. She died several weeks later. The memory of this event has never left me, and, even worse, a miserable fear for the most harmless pup has persisted."[2] It seems that a pathological association is welded between an emotion of fear and the terrifying situation that produced it. As a result of the human tendency to generalize when similar situations arise in the future the associated fear arises with them. So out of a single object causing the original fear, a phobia is extended to any number of similar objects or situations. Fortunately, as a result of this generalization one does not have to cure one after another all the various objects feared. If one gets rid of the fear of one of the objects in the group the patient will be immune to fear arising from all others.[3]

In the phobias we have just been considering, the patient remembers the incident from which they developed or if the incident has been forgotten the unreasonable fear is not of recent origin. But sometimes the incident that caused the phobia took place many years ago and then only later in life an anxiety develops that seems to have no motivation whatsoever.

In these cases one will often be able to demonstrate that the patient was well adjusted and happy from early life or until he was involved in a very unhappy situation, one that he did not want to face or even to acknowledge its existence. This resulted in maladjustment to his present surroundings and abiding unhappiness and discontent. The patient does not want to face the real cause of his anxiety but refers it to something that has an association with an emotional shock in early life. Again the cause that the patient picks out as the cause of his anxiety may be something in the present. In the war neuroses, for instance, anxiety states were referred to the possibility of someone being dead at home, whereas, the real cause was the fear that somebody might be killed in France.

---

[2] John Edward Wallace Wallin. *Minor Mental Maladjustments in Normal People.* Durham, N.C., 1939, p. 40.
[3] The first experimental study of the origin of fears in children seems to have been John B. Watson's and Rosalie Rayner's "Conditioned Emotional Reactions," *J. Exp. Psychol.* 1920. Watson's work seems to negate Frink's principle "What" the patient fears is his own unconscious sexual impulses. H. W. Frink *Morbid Fears and Compulsions.* New York, 1918, p. 433. On the treatment of fears see: Arthur T. Jersild and Frances Baker Holmes *Children's Fears.* New York, Bureau of Publications, Teachers College, Columbia University, 1935 and Mary Coover Jones *J. Exp. Psychol.*, 1924, pp. 382-390.

3. Self Treatment of Phobias and Major Mental Difficulties

We may now raise the question whether or not it is always necessary
to have expert psychiatric assistance in overcoming one's own abnormal
fear reactions. The answer is: No. One can force himself to carry on
and act normally in spite of intense unreasonable fear. The same is
true of fear that has a solid basis in the danger of the present moment
on the field of battle.

When anyone suffers from a phobia, he should know that if he is
willing to browbeat his unreasonable fear and will do so perseveringly
and allow no exceptions it will finally fade away and disappear. A
man once told me that when a boy he had seen a trolley wire break
and someone was killed by contact with the live wire. After that he
became intensely fearful whenever he had to pass under a trolley wire.
Eventually in order to get to his home he had to pass along an unpaved
street through which trolley cars returned to the barn. Though not
directly under the trolley wires, he feared that one might break and
swing over to where he walked and kill him. It is said that Mark
Twain once remarked: "I have had many troubles in my life, but
most of them never happened."

He finally concluded that he was going to have a fight with his
phobia to the finish. So he went out and walked along the tracks
directly under the trolley wire not only to his house but all the way to
the barn and back again. It required great effort and he suffered
intensely but he won out. Reality gained the day and the phobia
disappeared.

Not only in minor mental disorders but even in major conditions
cure is possible without psychiatric assistance. A man once told me of
how he suffered from a complex of alcoholism, sadism, masochism,
fetishism, and homosexuality. He finally looked at himself squarely
in the face and realized that unless he got over his condition he would
certainly end his days in the penitentiary. God must have given him
generously of His illuminating and inspiring graces. He asked for
God's help and became a daily communicant. After excessive indulgence in alcohol for about 20 years, he became a total abstainer
and rid himself of his sexual abnormalities. I have known psychiatrists
who would have told him that he was incurable and had to settle down
to his abnormalities with prudent care.[4] The success of Alcoholics

---

[4] T. V. Moore, *Nature and Treatment of Mental Disorders*, 2nd Ed. New York, Grune
and Stratton, 1951, pp. 339-340.

Anonymous derives from their insistence on the appeal to God for help. In the phobias, sanctity might well manifest its fundamental incompatibility with mental disorder. Sanctity is associated with voluntary self-denial in association with the Passion of Christ for the welfare of mankind. One who has a phobia does not want to fight against it. It seems easier to worry. True sanctity would arouse the patient to action. There could be no more wholesome self-denial for him than suffering entailed by carrying on bravely without yielding to the compulsion of the phobia. And the result would inevitably be emotional freedom. And as we have just seen sanctity contends successfully with conditions far more serious than phobias.

4. Advantage-Seeking Reactions

We shall now study an example of the advantage-seeking adjustments to the problems of life. Let us commence at once with an illustration.

During the First World War the author was a psychiatrist in the Medical Corps of the United States Army and was stationed at a little hospital near Verdun. When one was officer of the day and an engagement was going on, he could expect at any time of the night or day one or more ambulances conveying what was commonly termed "shell-shocked" soldiers. This term was forbidden in the army and such soldiers were said to be suffering from a *war neurosis*.

I recall to mind one night when as officer of the day I was awakened and went to a rather dimly lighted, relatively large hut. Soldiers were being brought in: some on stretchers still wet with bright red stains of blood from carrying the wounded in an engagement still going on. Apparently some soldiers with violent leg tremors could not walk. The wounded were not sent to us.

The patients were seated on benches and made a remarkable sight with the bizarre shaking of arms and legs. The instructions were to cure the tremors before putting the patients to bed. I was surprised to find out that this was nearly always not only possible but easy. Only rarely did one put a patient to bed who held on to his tremor. He was then put to bed but screened off from everyone. The result was that his tremors disappeared in a few days. The psychiatrists held that this was not so much due to rest in bed as to the fact that in an "hysterical" patient what cannot be seen evokes no sympathy and is not worth having.

A word about the technique of treatment. It was based on the fact that a relaxed muscle cannot tremble and you can relax the muscles of arm or leg by repeated, fairly rapid bending to and fro at the joints. . You would do this, say with a shaking arm, and finally "shake out" the hand and the whole arm would hang limp and the patient would look at his arm aghast to see that his defense reaction against duty at the front was gone completely. You would then say: Take your seat. Next. And start on the next man. Should a "cured" patient on the—— bench start to shake again, you would call out "Stop that"; step over and give a few more relaxations and return to your patient on the floor. When you had "cured" all, you would send them to bed. The next morning they were a happy lot. But they were not returned at once to the front. At a staff meeting it was decided after studying them for a while whether to send them back to their "outfit" or return them to the United States. I remember a New York policeman who said to me: "Captain, I can't stand those big guns. If you send me back I will simply break down again."

Besides tremors there were cases of emotional blindness, deafness and dumbness (aphonia). The validity of the army diagnosis of these cases as forms of hysteria, evasions of danger when on duty, was brilliantly illustrated on the day of the armistice. Except for a few exceptions, all in our little hospital of some 300 patients were clamoring to be returned to duty. The few exceptions had been falsely diagnosed in the confusion of battle. Thus one soldier was sent back as a case of "shell shock" because he fainted from time to time. He had typhoid and fainted from intestinal hemorrhage.

These cases illustrate the advantage-seeking reactions to the difficulties of life. The "hysterical" disability has a value in the mind of the patient. It is an evasion of danger that there is a moral duty to face and to accept its consequence.

Seeing that we are speaking of sanctity and insanity let us ask would a patient leading a good solid devout spiritual life be as likely to be diverted into an evasion of duty as one who might be entirely lacking in anything like a spiritual life?

Let us here consider the inner life of a poet soldier in France: Joyce Kilmer.

In view of the fact that some maintain that no war is justifiable a few remarks on the ethics of war and the problem that confronted the United States at the outbreak of the First World War will be necessary to appreciate the religious idealism of Kilmer.

The end and purpose of all government is to help the citizens to organize and develop their country to an extent which would be impossible to unorganized private enterprise; and to give them security in the pursuit of life, liberty and happiness by defending them against aggression. When the very existence of the commonwealth is threatened the men in authority in the government would sin if they were false to the trust they had assumed. The citizens of the commonwealth in their turn have a duty to offer their services to the government in its defense of the commonwealth.

In defending the commonwealth the government must exercise all possible prudence. It would not be wise to wait until the aggressor was at the door before taking steps against him. At the time of the First World War it was held by many that the German Empire had commenced a war destined to conquer Europe and the world. There were solid grounds for such a conviction. It was felt that if the United States did not enter the war against Germany with the Allies, we would soon have to fight a much more powerful Germany single handed. On the basis of such considerations the United States declared war.

Joyce Kilmer was one of those who believed that the freedom of the world was at stake and left his wife and children to offer his life in defense of man's right to serve God and live in accordance with Christian ideals. Only from that point of view can his life and poetry be understood. We present this religious attitude of mind as something that is a powerful antidote to the evasive disabilities of the war neuroses. Sound spirituality is in many ways incompatible with a number of mental disorders.

We get a picture of the daily religious life of Joyce Kilmer from a letter he wrote while at the front: "Pray that I may love God more. It seems to me that if I can learn to love God more passionately, more constantly without distractions, that absolutely nothing else can matter. Except while we are in the trenches I receive Holy Communion every morning, so it ought to be all the easier for me to attain this object of my prayers. I got Faith, you know, by praying for it. I hope to get Love the same way."[5]

And so Joyce Kilmer prayed that he might love God more

---

[5] *Joyce Kilmer*, ed. with *Memoir* by Robert Cortes Holliday. New York, G. H. Doran, Vol. I, p. 101. Letter to Sr. Mary Emerentia of St. Joseph's College, Toronto Ontario.

passionately, more constantly without distractions on the battlefields
of the First World War. It was something ever on his mind. In
another letter he asked: "Pray for me, my dear Father, that I may
love God more and that I may be unceasingly conscious of Him—that
is the greatest desire I have."[6]

This complete consecration to the Divine Will and the answer to his
prayer to be unceasingly conscious of the Divine Presence was the
source of his cool bravery on all occasions. Death did not matter.
Father Duffy, the chaplain of his regiment said of him: "He was
absolutely the coolest and most indifferent man in the face of danger I
have ever seen." The unseen presence of Divinity did not forsake him
in the hour of duty. And so he wrote, with no mere poetic figure of
speech, but with all the reality of one who had enjoyed in some manner
the mystic experience:

> Who fights for Freedom, goes with joyful tread,
> To meet the fires of Hell against him hurled
> And has for Captain Him whose thorn wreathed head,
> Smiles from the Cross upon a conquered world.

And then there were the days of long marches with the heavy pack
and the hand that was numbed with cold while it held the rifle. There
were those who grumbled and complained and swore in their chill wet
clothing. But to Kilmer it was a time for prayer and union with
Christ in His Passion. And so he gave his mind to meditation and
lived in union with Christ in his sufferings. And the following poem is
the outline of the meditation of this soldier in France.

> My shoulders ache beneath my pack
> (Lie easier Cross upon His back).
> I march with feet that burn and smart
> (Tread, Holy Feet, upon my heart).
> Men shout at me who may not speak
> (They scourged Thy back and smote Thy cheek).
> I may not lift a hand to clear
> My eyes of salty drops that sear.
> Then shall my fickle soul forget
> Thy agony of Bloody Sweat?

---

[6] Letter to Father Garesche, S. J., op. cit., Vol. II, p. 119.

> My rifle hand is stiff and numb
> (From Thy pierced palm red rivers come).
> So let me render back again
> This millionth of Thy gift.   Amen.

A life with God before he enlisted in the army in the cause of freedom was the beginning of a spiritual growth which attained its heights during his service at the front. One day when overwhelmed by almost hopeless difficulties he sat down and wrote his poem of thanksgiving: a cry of the faith and confidence of a soul that lives with God.

> The roar of the world is in my ears
> Thank God for the roar of the world,
> Thank God for the mighty tide of fears
> Against me always hurled.
> Thank God for the bitter and ceaseless strife,
> And the sting of His chastening rod!
> Thank God for the stress and pain of life,
> And oh, thank God for God!

It was natural and fitting that the heroic sanctity of this common soldier in France should be crowned by civic martyrdom on the field of battle.

The life and poems of Joyce Kilmer take the soul beyond the point where all psychiatry must end. They deliver the troubled mind to Him Who said:

> Fear not for I have redeemed thee and called thee
> by thy name. Thou art Mine.
> When thou shalt pass through the waters, I will be
> with thee, and the rivers shall not cover thee;
> When thou shalt walk in the fire, thou shalt not be
> burnt, and the flames shall not consume thee.
> For I am the Lord, thy God, the Holy One of Israel,
> thy Savior. (Isaias XLIII:1-3).

CHAPTER XVII

St. Thérèse and the Problem of Emotional Control*

1. Abnormal Irritability

If we designate by the word *irritability* a general tendency to cause trouble in all social contacts we have a common trait in a number of normal people. It seems to be an element of some value in the prognosis of a major mental breakdown and many conditions which are usually classified under personality disorders.

From the purely physiological point of view it may be regarded at times as a defective inhibition by the cerebral cortex of the emotional centers in the midbrain. Thus in dogs, in which the cortex has been separated from the thalamic region, every stimulus leads to what looks like a violent outbreak of rage. One can perhaps understand this by considering what is termed an exaggerated knee jerk. There are two neurons (nerve cells with their fibres) that go (1) from the motor cortex in the brain to the spinal cord (2) from the spinal cord to the muscle. When both neurons are intact a tap on the tendon of the knee leads to a slight kicking movement known as the knee jerk. But if the upper motor neuron is severed there is a much exaggerated kick or perhaps a rhythmic series of jerks. The upper motor neuron must, therefore, tone down the activity of the lower motor neurons.

In the same way there are emotional centers in the midbrain. Electrical stimulation of the hypothalamus in man[1] and manipulation

---

*In the present work we make use of St. Thérèse of Lisieux along with other saints to illustrate sanctity. We also show that there is no ground for the charge made against her that she was a psychopath who had a mental breakdown. The psychologist and psychiatrist will find in this chapter an empirical study of the psychology of religion in childhood.

[1] Roy R. Grinker and Herman M. Serota. "Studies on Corticohypothalamic Relations in the Cat and Man", *J. Neurophysio.* 1936, *1,* 573-589.

of the hypothalamus in operations[2] arouse various types of emotional experience.

Mental disorders arising from cortical destruction are associated at times with an appearance of irritability and other emotional symptoms. We can understand this as a loss of inhibition due to injury to the "upper neurons."[3] After "encephalitis," children are prone to violent outbreaks of temper. In the gradual increase of destruction of cortical tissue due to repeated tiny cortical hemorrhages in arteriosclerosis, and also in aging, there may come on a gradual change of character. Impatience, which had long disappeared from the patient's life, and later angry episodes, a tendency to murmur, criticize, and be antagonistic to others present new problems for self-control.

If man were an organism used by the brain there could be no modification in the progress of hypermotivity due to vascular disorders. But man is a being who uses the brain to manage himself and adjust himself to the varied problems of life. Consequently, if the progress of cortical destruction is sufficiently slow man can use other pathways to control emotions just as a telephone operator can connect one city with another by using one of several possible lines when a falling tree in a thunderstorm cuts off one line of communication. And so even post-encephalitic children with temper tantrums can be reeducated to normal behavior.

2. Abnormal Conduct and Brain Disorder

If one studies the encephalogram[4] of early adolescents who are diagnosed as having a personality disorder, one will be able to divide them into two groups: (a) those whose encephalograms are normal and (b) those in whom waves appear indicative of organic cerebral pathology. Some behavior disorders are due to lack of ideals and voluntary control; in others the steering gear is broken.

We must not, however, draw the conclusion that adolescents,

---

[2] W. E. LeGros Clark et alii, *The Hypothalamus*, Edinburgh, Oliver and Boyd, 1938, p. 117.

[3] See hereon Jean Delay, *Les dérèglements de l'humeur*, Paris, Presses Universitaires de France, 1946.

[4] An encephalogram is a tracing obtained from an instrument known as an encephalograph. By putting pairs of electrodes at various regions on the head changes in potential in the underlying cerebral tissue appear as undulations in the encephalogram.

suffering from organic cerebral pathological conditions, are all hopeless cases and it is vain to treat them. For remember that man uses his brain, it is not the brain that uses the man. We may well expect to have greater difficulty with the pathological problems. These cases resemble those termed constitutional psychopathic inferiority. But if a good psychiatrist succeeds in establishing a friendly rapport with such a child, there is solid ground on which to base hope of making over its character.

If we ask ourselves what causes disorders of the personality in a patient when there is no injury to the brain, due for instance to "sleeping sickness" called *encephalitis lethargica,* we naturally look for defects of training in an inadequate home. They can often be demonstrated.

Now here is where we come to another type of incompatibility between sanctity and mental disorder. There can be no perfect sanctity without full control of emotional manifestations. One who has not the ideal of perfect conformity to the will of God might make no effort to preserve or regain the emotional control that he saw gradually disappearing from his life. In this case, as cortical destruction increased, his difficulties with those about him would multiply and he would gradually pass into some mental condition such as arteriosclerosis associated with "behavioral reaction."

In like manner, if an individual with congenital weakness of inhibition of the hypothalamus by the cortex, never attempted in developmental years to strengthen personal emotional control, he would develop a personality disorder which would be classified as some form of "personality trait disturbance" or "sociopathic personality disturbance."

3. Did St. Thérèse Suffer from Brain Disorder?

It is in this field of inadequate emotional control that evidence has been looked for to support the contention that St. Thérèse was a "neuropath." The etymology of neuropath gives it the sense of one suffering from brain disorder. Seeing however that children in general suffer from more or less inadequate emotional control, the crucial problem is: Was the emotional control of St. Thérèse pathologically defective *throughout childhood and later life?*

Father Robo's accusations. Father Etienne Robo's accusations against St. Thérèse may thus be summarized.

1. She was a spoiled child.[5]
2. Her childhood faults "were not manifestations of her real character and we cannot attach any importance to them. What counted was this: that she had a very tender, abnormally tender, conscience which made her pathetically unhappy until she had been able to confess her baby sins to her mother and obtained forgiveness."[6]
3. After her mother's death "she became timid, retiring and so sensitive 'that a look,' she says, 'was enough to make me burst into tears.'[7] Pauline's care and solicitude had little or no effect on the new morbid sensitiveness, the timidity, the brooding that had changed the child's character suddenly after her mother's death."[8]
4. "She liked solitude, and at the age of six, seven, eight would retire by herself 'to think of *eternity*,' She is 'an exile'; she 'longs for the repose of heaven.' At the age of six this is less a sign of religious fervor than one of a morbid tendency to melancholy. When we read of the constantly recurring black moods of her later years, of her scruples, of her doubts, we are confirmed in this opinion."[9]
5. "She was just over twelve when, before her second communion in 1885, she began to be tormented by scruples, and this went on for at least eight years and possibly much longer."[10]
6. "Since her mother's death she had always cried easily, this tendency was if anything intensified as she grew up."[11]
7. "At school where she was sent when she was about nine, she was a quiet child who disliked games and stood apart from the other girls. She preferred reading or thinking. 'During recreation I frequently gave myself up to serious thoughts while from a distance I watched my companions play. . . .' At home during the holidays she often hid herself in a corner of her room behind the bed curtains and there 'I thought of God, the brevity of life and eternity.' " [11a]

---

[5] *Two Portraits*, 2nd Ed., Westminster, Md., Newman, p. 57.
[6] Loc. cit., p. 64.
[7] Loc. cit., p. 66.
[8] Loc. cit., p. 66.
[9] Loc. cit., p. 73.
[10] Loc. cit., p. 74, this is not true according to St. Thérèse's account as we shall see.
[11] Loc. cit., p. 75.
[11a] Loc. cit., pp. 75-76.

To put all this briefly we may list the charges as follows:

1. She was a spoiled child.
2. She had an over-tender conscience and was scrupulous.
3. She had a tendency to sadness and a desire to be alone.
4. She developed an abnormal tearfulness.

To what extent are these charges true and do they mean a mental disorder? Let us see.

Was St. Thérèse a spoiled child? What is understood by a spoiled child? Children are spoiled when intense affection for a child makes a parent blind to the duty of regulating that affection so as to give due attention to wise and wholesome limitations of a child's deviations from right conduct. There need be no limit to parental affection in order to train a child, so long as the parent does not allow himself or herself to be blinded by affection to the welfare of the child. A spoiled child is disobedient and subject to tantrums.

Was St. Thérèse allowed by her parents and sisters to do what she pleased without restraint? Did she develop the spirit of disobedience characteristic of spoiled children, along with the tantrums, that spoiled children manifest if one attempts to insist upon obedience? Father Robo's statement that Thérèse was a spoiled child seems to have been arrived at hastily without considering important available evidence.

It is true that St. Thérèse was loved with a tender and intense affection by her father. But did that lead him to let her have her own way without restraint and become a disobedient child given to angry tantrums? A former housemaid in M. Guérin's home, afterwards a Benedictine nun, gave the following testimony in the Canonical Process about Mr. Martin's training of his favorite little child.

"The Servant of God, Thérèse, whom he called his 'little Queen,' being the youngest, was the object of his special affection, but this did not lessen in any way the serious tone of his education of her. He would not tolerate any fault in her. Without being severe, he raised his children in fidelity to all their duties."[12]

Sister Genevieve (Céline), at her deposition at the Apostolic Process, told how Mr. Martin reproached little Thérèse and scolded her so severely for not having yielded to her elder sister that Céline herself was extremely upset.[13]

---

[12](Sister Genevieve of the Holy Face). *The Father of the Little Flower*. Trans. by Rev. Michael Collins, Westminster, Md., Newman, 1955, p. 44.

[13]Op. cit., p. 45.

At meals "there was no making of faces or showing repugnance if one did not like a dish. 'No soup, no meat.' "[14]

There are some important facts in an article on *Pauline* by the Rev. F. Horsfield.[15]

"Teresa had been out for a long walk on a hot summer day and came home very tired and thirsty; 'Give me a drink, Pauline, please' she called as she came into the house. 'A good chance to make a sacrifice,' suggested Pauline. Teresa was silent for a moment, then smiled bravely, trying hard and indeed succeeding in doing as her big sister said. When Pauline saw that the sacrifice had indeed been willingly made, she told Teresa to go and get herself a glass of lemonade. 'But what about my sacrifice?' objected Teresa. 'You've already won the merit of that' Pauline answered, 'now you will get the merit of obedience as well.' And on the top of both she got the glass of lemonade."[16]

The article continues: "The saint recalls 'how you (Pauline) often used to send me by myself at night to fetch things from a room at the other side of the house, wisely taking no refusal; it was really good for me because I was far too timid. Now it is very hard to frighten me. It is a wonder to me how you managed to bring me up so lovingly without spoiling me, but you certainly did. You never let me off with a single little fault and never went back on any decision that you made, though you never rebuked me unless there was good cause!' Many years later, Pauline, now Mother Agnes of Jesus, gave her impressions on this point saying: 'Teresa spoke of the way in which I brought her up. But I reproach myself for certain severities, which were useless for this little one from heaven.' "[17]

From the incident about the lemonade we see the secret of Pauline's success in training St. Thérèse. It was an appeal to the religious value of sacrifice. As she grew older she saw that little sacrifices buy souls for Christ. So in the trials of obedience she made her sacrifice and gave up her own way for the love of Christ.

Here we can see how striving for the perfection of sanctity introduces an incompatibility with the development of a psychoneurotic character defect such as disobedience and tantrums. The disorder is cured in its

---

[14]Op. cit., p. 48.
[15]*The Saint of Liseux*, July, 1952, *9*, pp. 48-52.
[16]Loc. cit., p. 49.
[17]Loc. cit., pp. 49-50.

beginnings by a psychotherapy that eliminates character defects and develops a stable personality. In this development it is not mere strength of will that carries off the victory, but rather religious ideals. These are not merely ordinary concepts of the mind but the activity of God's illuminating grace and the natural strength of the will is fortified by God's inspiring grace. But of these factors Father Robo seems to have no inkling. *All* human activity, according to him, derives from a driving power due to unreasoned instincts that lurk in the dim recesses of the *unconscious*![18]

A tender conscience and scrupulosity. The tender conscience of St. Thérèse in childhood was perhaps a gift of God which was given her in the light of His Knowledge that she would cooperate with Him and never commit a mortal sin in all her life. It led to what we may term a *sense of sin.* A sense of sin is the power to understand what it means to deliberately reject the God of Infinite Love in order to enjoy some finite creature. Along with this realization there comes a strong vibrant resonance throughout the body after one has sinned. Thus when Our Lord turned and looked on Peter, just after he had cursed and sworn that he knew Him not, Peter realized the enormity of his crime; and going out he wept bitterly.

It is perfectly true that the love of God and true sorrow for sin are in themselves pure acts of the will, turning to God and away from sin. But that does not mean that these pure acts of the will have no resonance in the body. And so, since man is *one* substance and *not two*—a body and a soul, each a distinct substance—a resonance in the body can flow from an intellectual realization.[19]

St. Thérèse's tears for her petty faults in childhood did her no harm. But they prepared her to understand more fully the meaning of the Love of God and the sins of men as her knowledge of the Faith developed. The resulting sense of sin helped her to be faithful to her Eternal Spouse all through her life.

Children fall often into objective sin before they understand what sin is and what it means. Therefore, they easily sin later with adequate

---

[18] *The Two Portraits*, 2nd ed. pp. 78-79. Father Robo makes no use of Stephane-Joseph Piat. *The Story of a Family.* Trans. by Benedictine of Stanbrook Abbey. New York, Kenedy, 1948. Piat produces many facts that make it impossible to hold that St. Thérèse was a spoiled child. No spoiled child is obedient at home and at school throughout childhood. See Chapters IX, XI, XII.

[19] St. Thomas Aquinas: *Summa Theologica.* 1. 2. Q. XXXV, i.

knowledge and consent. But had a home like that of St. Thérèse developed within them a true sense of sin and fidelity to the God of Love, they might have attained to sanctity by the way of innocence. There is no essential connection between a sense of sin and the origin of scrupulosity. Scrupulosity originates most frequently around the age of adolescence. (See page 8). The reason for this is not known. Almost a half of 400 high school girls had suffered from a passing attack of scruples.[19a] It would seem that scrupulosity is ordinarily nothing more than a parataxis of anxiety. (See page 127).

At times, but rarely, it is associated with something distinctly pathological: a compulsion. For example, a drive to look at a holy picture and then a drive to look at it again and again accompanied by the thought: I will commit a mortal sin if I don't look. Such phenomena would indicate that something more serious than a parataxis might be in the offing.

The scruples of St. Thérèse seem not to have had anything to do with her normal "sense of sin" that kept her from mortal sin all her life. They came on suddenly in May 1885 during the retreat for the solemn renewal of her First Communion. They constituted a severe trial. When her sister Marie entered Carmel in October 1886 she lost the only one to whom she could mention her absurd anxieties. In her desperation she prayed to her four little brothers and sisters who died in infancy.[20] "The answer was not long in coming; soon my soul was flooded with the sweetest peace."[21] The duration of the period of constant intense scrupulosity was about one year and a half. The intense chronic anxiety cleared. But from time to time afterwards her judgment was clouded and the old anxiety returned, to be dissipated by talking things over with a confessor.

There is no evidence that St. Thérèse was incapacitated by these anxieties. (See above, p. 129). At the height of her scrupulosity she carried on her studies and stood well in her classes or was a gentle obedient pupil with Madame Papinau. A psychoneurosis, as we have seen is regarded as a partial defect of temperament which involves some degree of incapacitation. St. Thérèse was tormented by her

[19a]J. J. Mullen, Psychological Factors in the Pastoral Treatment of Scruples. Stud. Psychol. and Psychiat. *I*, 1927.

[20]F. J. Sheed, *Collected Letters*. Sheed and Ward, 1949, p. 14, also Autobiography, Chapter IV.

[21]Autobiography, Taylor's translation, p. 69. *Manuscript* 44 right.

scrupulosity while it lasted—about a year and a half. It was not associated with any genuine pathological condition as a compulsion. She was outstanding in her ability to get along with others all her life.

Like everyone else St. Thérèse had her mental trials, but she endured them patiently for the love of God without developing anything that can be diagnosed as a definite type of mental disorder. Great scrupulosity is mentioned by Benedict XIV among the trials to which the saints are subjected.

The sadness of St. Thérèse and her desire to be all alone. St. Thérèse does write of her *sadness* after her mother's death. It was indeed genuine deep sadness. But it was not the pathological sadness that never lifts: that comes on when one awakes in the morning and hangs on in deep gloom throughout the day. The picture we have of her general mood, from independent sources and that of her letters of the period, is that of a gay and happy child enjoying life with her sisters and cousins with intense delight.

Thus Mrs. Guérin writes shortly after the death of Thérèse's mother: "Thérèse's goodness simply enchants me . . . she will be delighted to see her father and sisters again, but she is gay, very gay, she laughs so heartily that she starts me laughing."[22]

She had her periods of sadness when she thought of her mother who had gone to heaven, but she passed with joy and laughter into the life of the day.

But how about that *morbid tendency to melancholy* when she went off to be alone and think of eternity; when she felt herself alone and longed for the repose of heaven?

One must recall again Father Robo's fundamental principle: "In the dim recesses of the unconscious lurk in us all some innate inclinations, unreasoned instincts. . . . They are the driving power behind all human activities, and lacking it we should lead the life of the sloth on his tree."[23]

On this principle it is impossible to understand human conduct, let alone the psychology of the saints in whom are realized Our Lord's words: "If any man love Me he will keep My word and My Father will love him and We will come to him and will make Our abode with him." (John XIV:23). The love of God is not an unreasoned instinct

---

[22]*Collected Letters of Saint Therese of Lisieux*, Trans. by F. J. Sheed, New York, Sheed and Ward, 1949, p. 9.

[23]*Two Portraits of St. Thérèsa of Lisieux*, Westminster, Md., Newman Press. Pp. 78-79.

but an act of free human responsibility flowing from an intellectual knowing due to divine grace sanctifying the soul, illuminating the intellect and inspiring the will. God Who makes His abode in the soul keeps His word. God and the soul live together in a pact of perfect and eternal friendship. This life of the soul with God commenced in St. Thérèse at a very early age. She was precocious both in her intellectual and in her spiritual development. Her life with God was not, as Father Robo says, a morbid tendency to melancholy. No man can be understood without realizing that he has an intellect that transcends all animal intelligence and that his responsible conduct is a free act in the conscious light of ideals and concepts that intellect alone can conceive.

When St. Thérèse went to school this same precocious development of her spiritual life drew her to Him Who had made His abode within her. This was something altogether different from a precox withdrawal. It was no more a shut-in type of reaction than the gathering of readers around the lights in a library is a mere mechanical tropism such as is manifested in unicellular organisms, and termed a phototaxis.

St. Thérèse was not the only child who ever wanted to be all alone with God. There was a little Irish girl, Nellie Organ, whose mother died of tuberculosis when Nellie was 3 years and 5 months old. A few months later she was taken to the orphanage of the Good Shepherd Sisters at Sunday's Well, Cork. A little later it was found that Little Nellie of Holy God, as she is now known, was suffering from an advanced condition of tuberculosis.

In some way, without any special instruction by anyone, she developed a deep knowledge of God and the mystery of the Holy Eucharist. She lived in "almost unbroken spiritual communion with Holy God."[24] She used to ask the nurse to come back to her right after receiving holy communion and kiss her and then return and make her thanksgiving. Having received the kiss she would wave her hand for her to go back to the chapel, but would never say a word so as not to disturb the nurse's thanksgiving.[25]

A Jesuit priest obtained permission for her to make her first Holy Communion. She thereafter prepared herself for holy communion

---

[24]This and the other data and quotations are derived from Maire Cotter *Little Nellie of Holy God*. Dublin, Clonmore and Reynolds, 1956, p. 35.
[25]P. 36.

by retiring into herself the night before "thinking about Holy God and talking to Holy God." In the morning she kept perfect silence. "So that her adoration would not be disturbed (after communion) by outward distraction, she would sometimes ask to be turned towards the wall. Very often her thanksgiving lasted for three hours, and once it continued until late in the evening. Of that occasion a Sister writes: 'When I visited her about a quarter to five in the evening, she was lying quite still in her little cot, turned towards the window. I had heard of her strange condition during the day, and was very curious to see her. I bent over her, and as I did so, Nellie turned suddenly and said: "Oh Mudder, I'm so happy. I've been talking to Holy God." Her voice trembled with delight, her face, previously so dusky with the ravages of disease, was now white as milk. Her cheeks glowed (I can best express what I mean by saying) 'as a smiling peach.' Her large eyes shone with such brilliancy that one could not help thinking: These eyes have seen God. Her smile cannot be described because it was of heaven, and around the bed was a distinct aroma of incense."[26]

God has given us for our instruction this example of a child in its fourth year who had an unsurpassed realization of the mystery of the Eucharist and who lived without interruption in the Divine Omnipresence.

Father Robo says of St. Thérèse's retiring into herself at the age of 6, 7, 8 to think of eternity and long for heaven that "this is less a sign of religious fervor than one of a morbid melancholy."[27] But here again he is reading his own mind into the conduct of St. Thérèse and not deriving his opinion from objective evidence. When Little Nellie of Holy God, after a day spent in thanksgiving for receiving Our Lord, said: "O Mudder, I'm so happy. I've been talking to Holy God," she was certainly not suffering from melancholy. Neither Little Nellie nor St. Thérèse in their quest of solitude were yielding to a schizophrenic shut-in reaction, a drive to get away from men, but following God's call to be alone with Him and commune with Him in the indescribable joy of His Presence.[28]

---

[26]Pp. 45-46. Various witnesses attest similar observations.

[27]*The Two Portraits*, p. 73.

[28]Nineteen months after the child's death, the grave was opened in the presence of witnesses, before removing it from the cemetary to the convent. The body was found intact except for a small cavity in the right jaw from which (caries) the child suffered when living. The fingers were quite flexible. Everything in the coffin was exactly as it was when she was buried.

Tearfulness. The best picture of the tearfulness of St. Thérèse is given by herself in the fourth chapter of her autobiography.

At the time of Marie's entrance into Carmel "I was much given to crying, not only over big things, but over trifling ones too. For instance: I was anxious to advance in virtue but I went about it in a strange way. I was not accustomed to wait on myself;[29] Céline always arranged our room, and I never did any housework. Sometimes in order to please Our Lord, I used to make my bed, or, if she were out in the evening, to bring in her plants and seedlings. As I said before it was simply to please Our Lord that I did these things, and so I ought not to have expected any thanks from creatures.[30] But, alas, I did expect them, and if unfortunately Céline did not seem surprised and grateful for my little service, I was not pleased, and tears rose to my eyes.

"Again if by accident I offended anyone, instead of taking it in the right way, I fretted till I made myself ill, thus making my fault worse, instead of mending it; and when I began to realize my foolishness, I would cry for having cried."[31]

Are we to look upon this tendency to cry as due to an organic condition such as described in the beginning of this chapter: an anatomical defect of the pathway from the hypothalamus to the cortex or rather to underlying mental factors?

The actually existing mental factors and also the suddenness with which Thérèse overcame her tendency to cry indicate that the mental trials that Thérèse underwent since her mother's death might well have caused an abiding fretfulness that made it easy for her to cry.

The fundamental condition arose from her mother's death. Then Pauline became her mother; but soon Pauline entered Carmel. Then Marie became her mother; and a little later Marie entered Carmel.

---

[29]This whole part of the chapter has been rearranged and abbreviated. The original preludes this sentence with the words "Since I was the last child." The strange condition had developed from Thérèse being spared housework by her older sisters because she was so little. See Manuscript p. 45, left, top.

[30]This expectancy is very pronounced in women. Men in general do not appreciate that a woman always expects thanks for little things. I once said Mass at a convent for a number of consecutive days. Every morning there was a prettily arranged centerpiece of flowers that I did not even notice. One morning, to my surprise, the Sister who served burst out indignantly. "If those pansies would jump up and bow and say good morning you would not be surprised".

[31]Taylor's translation *Soeur Thérèse of Lisieux*, New York, Kenedy, 1924, pp. 68-69.

When Léonie was with the Visitation nuns or the Poor Clares, Céline and Thérèse were left alone with their father. They were witnessing the dissolution of that wonderfully happy home of which memories alone remained. A poet's words of the autumn seem to describe the home of Thérèse at this period. "Now fretful whine the gusts through barren tree and vine."

Something similar happens to children who at a mother's death are placed by the Department of Charities first in one home then in another, rendering impossible the permanent fixation of a child's love on any "mother." St. Thérèse was also undergoing in childhood what is the normal lot of those who live to see the home die in old age. It was a severe mental burden to which she reacted, not a neurological organic defect of emotional control.

She tells us that she tried her best to get over her tearfulness but could not: "all reasoning was impossible, I could not correct myself of this ugly fault."[32] What made things worse, she felt she could not enter Carmel as a cry baby.

God answers our prayers and gives His help in due season when perhaps, we least expect it. His answer came Christmas night 1886 a little before Thérèse was fourteen years of age (January 2, 1887).

From earliest infancy, on returning from the midnight Mass she would find her shoes in the chimney corner. Her cries of delight at each little surprise were such a joy to the family that no one ventured to quit putting out the magic shoes when Christmas Eve rolled around again. But when Mr, Martin was going up stairs this time, Thérèse heard him say: "Really all this is too babyish for a big girl like Thérèse, and I hope it is the last year it will happen." "His words cut me to the quick. Céline knowing how sensitive I was whispered: 'Don't go down stairs just yet—wait a little, you would cry too much if you looked at your presents before Papa.' "

But she did and gave her dear King the last of those happy Christmas Eves that he was to enjoy on earth. "Céline thought she must be dreaming, but happily it was a reality; little Thérèse had regained, once for all the strength of mind which she had lost at the age of four and a half."[33]

Rightly does St. Thérèse attribute the change to divine grace. She

---

[32]Manuscript 45, left lines 16-17.
[33]Taylor's translation. P. 72.

ST. THÉRÈSE AND EMOTIONAL CONTROL 163

was now ready to enter Carmel. She would indeed cry again under severe provocation. But she did not shed a tear when all were sobbing as she entered Carmel. And in the convent she remained the valiant woman of Carmel who opened her mouth to wisdom; and in her life and writings has led souls along the way of sanctity.

From the dawn of her vocation at two years of age, she sought God without ceasing. She triumphed over all obstacles to her early entrance into Carmel. She bore her own defects with patience in the spirit of prayer. She was ever outstanding in her kind and loving relations to others. Her tearfulness which is pointed out as a neurotic trait was due to heavy sorrows weighing down on the mind of a child. But in all she was never a neurotic but by the grace of God a strong and vigorous personality.

Chapter XVIII

Sanctity and Organic Mental Disease

So far we have been dealing with mental disorders in which the experiences of life constituted an important contributing factor to their development. Or at least their appearance was not dependent on any clearly defined physical cause.

But there is another large group of mental disorders whose origin is found in one or more of the various ways in which the brain can suffer some kind of physical damage.

Thus an infectious disease or toxic substance inhaled or taken in to the system by the mouth or a blow or other injury to the head or any kind of cause, that produces more or less damage to the brain, can cause mental symptoms. When these symptoms are severe and more than transient duration they are grouped under the name of the *organic psychoses.*

Some of these conditions, though severe, nevertheless clear completely. The damage to the brain is said to be reversible. Others never clear; the damage is said to be irreversible. We might think, and in general it was thought in the recent past that the previous temperament or character of the individual would have nothing whatever to do with the symptoms due to organic brain disorder. But recent experience teaches us otherwise: "In all these reactions stemming from impairment of the function of the brain tissue, there are certain symptoms due to the structural change in the nerve cells, and others due to the patient's earlier experience and his habitual pattern of reaction to the world. Symptoms due to the impairment of brain-tissue function may be found in any age in life, beginning with birth injuries and terminating with the changes of senility."[1]

1. Acute Brain Disorders

Let us consider only one of the various types of mental disorders due to *acute* involvements of the cerebral tissues: *acute brain syndrome*

---

[1] J. R. Ewalt, E. A. Strecker and F. G. Ebaugh, *Practical Clinical Psychiatry*, Blakiston Division, McGraw-Hill, 8th Ed. New York, 1957, p. 101.

associated with systematic infection. Such disorders are not often seen in mental hospitals. Many last for only a few hours or days and are usually classified under the heading of the specific infection by which they were caused.

The common mental symptoms of all acute brain disorders are as follows:

A fluctuating impairment of consciousness. The patient may be perfectly clear at one period of the day and acutely confused at another. There are likely to be defects of memory. Thus in the afternoon the patient may accuse the physician of neglecting his morning visit because the fact of the visit has already faded from his memory.

As the condition develops *hallucinations* appear. They may arise *in all spheres of sensation* but auditory are more common. *Illusions,* that is false interpretations of real sensory objects, are frequently encountered. Both the hallucinations and the illusions are of a fear-producing type. *Delusions,* that is false interpretations of the conduct and intentions of others, are generally present.

The *behavior* of these patients is likely to be a reaction to their hallucinations: they run away, try to jump out of windows, or fall down stairs. Or they may be apparently stuporous in bed and again thrashing around and picking at the sheets.

The patient looks ill. "During the lucid intervals patients usually complain of headache and feelings of general weakness and debility."[2]

If the reader will consult the description we have given of the illness of St. Thérèse in her tenth year (below p. 213ff) he will recognize there the picture of this toxic mental reaction to some kind of an acute infectious disease.

There was an impairment of consciousness. Sometimes she recognized her relatives, sometimes she did not, as when she saw Marie and did not know who she was.

There were terrifying hallucinations. Her bed seemed surrounded by frightful precipices. There were illusions. "Nails in the wall took the form of terrifying appearances of long fingers, shrivelled and blackened with fire.

"One day, while Papa stood looking at me in silence, the hat in his

---

[2] Ewalt, Strecker and Ebaugh. *Practical Clinical Psychiatry.* p. 104. The above description of the general symptoms in "any toxic mental reaction" is drawn from this source.

hand was suddenly transformed into some horrible shape and I was so frightened that he went away sobbing."[3]

Father Robo himself speaks of her delusions. "At last she was under the delusion that the medicaments they gave her were poisonous. 'They want to poison me,' she cried."[4]

Father Robo calls attention to a passage in the original manuscript that was omitted in the redaction for the public. It reads thus: "But for a long time after my cure I believed that I had pretended on purpose to be sick, and that was a veritable martyrdom for my soul."[5] She spoke to her sister Marie about the matter and also to her confessor who pointed out to her that she never could have pretended all that she experienced. She says that God left her with this anxiety until she entered Carmel. The spiritual director at Carmel cleared her mind at once and completely.

It is strange that Father Robo does not recognize here one of her later scrupulosities on which he generally lays so much stress. We may take the opportunity to point out here another symptom in her illness which conforms to the picture of a mental condition depending on an acute infection: *the patient looks sick.* A healthy pretender could scarcely deceive a physician who along with her uncle decided that "she was suffering from a very serious illness such as he had never seen in a child so young."[6] Nor could a child of ten carry out in 1883 a drama of pretense which fitted symptom for symptom with the picture recognized today as "acute brain syndrome associated with systematic infection."

2. *Mental Symptoms in Acute and Chronic Brain Disorders*

Let us now turn to the picture of *chronic* brain disorders. As there are a group of symptoms common to all *acute* brain disorders, so also *chronic* brain disorders have their common symptoms.

In the brain itself there are organic changes that are irreversible.

---

[3] Taylor's translation of *Soeur Thérèse of Lisieux*, Kenedy, New York ninth impression, 1924, p. 49.

[4] The original manuscript merely says that they tried in vain to make her take "some very simple remedies". The reason why she refused was probably a delusion that they were poisoned. Such delusions are common in infectious deliria. Father Robo's account (*The Two Portraits*, p. 67) is based on Pere Petitot, O.P., pp. 105-107. Title of book not given.

[5] Manuscript p. 29 left.

[6] Manuscript p. 28 left.

In *acute* brain disorders one finds edema of the brain with swelling of the nerve cells and their supporting tissues. This condition may subside and recovery may be complete. Its reversals in the course of the illness might be conceived of as having something to do with the fluctuating impairment of consciousness noted in acute brain disorders. This fluctuation of the mental condition occurs also in some chronic brain disorders; but there are also permanent destructions of brain tissue with progressive mental impairment.

The mental impairment is found both in *cognitive* and *affective* conscious life. Cognitive defect is manifested in an inability to interpret sensory material, for example, to explain the evident meaning of a picture or the trend of meaning in a series of pictures such as found in the comic sheets of a newspaper. Affective disorder is manifested by intensity and unreasonableness of emotional display.

Von Monakow laid down the general principle that permanent defects of interpretation (agnosia) are never due to a local injury in a sound brain.[7] Whenever they are found, it points to diffuse impairment of the whole cortex. This is to be conceived of as essentially a sensory defect. Perception does not consist in a mere enumeration of sensory qualities but in the holding before the mind of a total picture that the mind can consider part by part without one part fading from consciousness when another is being considered. This ability of presenting the total picture is not merely that of the individual sense organ. For the sense organ may be perfectly intact and the presentation of all its data as a unit may be impossible. It is a special ability of what has been termed the *synthetic sense* and was known to Aristotle as the *sensus communis.*[8]

In what is termed the hypothalamic region of the brain there are reflex centers for emotional expression: the pounding of the heart, the heavy breathing, the drive to attack an enemy and many other resultants of any violent emotion. These centers when stimulated may give rise to intensified *conscious* emotional experience or an emotional resonance devoid of its usual type of awareness. Man's control of his emotional life is twofold: one *indirect* by turning his attention to other things till the emotion fades out; one *direct* by repressing emotional expression and a determination not to behave in that foolish way any

---

[7] C. von Monakow, *Die Lokalisation im Grosshirn*, Wiesbaden, 1914, p. 479.

[8] See hereon T. V. Moore *Cognitive Psychology*, Philadelphia, Lippincott; 1939. Part III, The Psychology of Perception, pp. 209-271.

longer. This control is psychic, not the mere physiological activity of
the cerebral cortex. But if the cerebral cortex is widely degenerated
or the connection between the cortex and the hypothalamic region is
seriously affected, that control can no more be exercised than the
driver of an automobile can direct it wherever he would, when the
steering gear is broken.

Sensory memory is also impaired in chronic brain disorders. It is
affected sometimes even prior to a noticeable involvement of the
synthetic sense with its presentation of the whole sensory picture.

With increasing weakening of emotional control, there comes on
eventually a profound change in the personality. When the prepsychotic personality was inadequate by reason of moral offenses,
irritability, antagonisms, quarreling, the deterioration of the personality is merely a gross exaggeration of its previous defects.

In some chronic brain disorders there is, as in acute conditions, a
fluctuation of certain symptoms.

Let us now consider senile dementia and arteriosclerosis.

3. Chronic Brain Syndrome Associated with Senile Brain Disease
In senile brain disease notable portions of the brain undergo
disintegration and absorption. This is evidenced by the fact that the
senile brain shows loss of weight. In addition there are areas of
softening and typical microscopic structures known as senile plaques.
"Recent work shows that these senile plaques occur with the same
frequency in non-psychotic old people as in those showing senile
mental changes, and the exact role such plaques play in the production
of symptoms is not clear.[9]

From the character of the cerebral changes we can understand that
the course of the disorder is long drawn out and progressive. In some
old people deterioration is more rapid than it need be by reason of a
faulty diet in what has been termed the "tea and toast" stage of
human life. Such people may have a remission due to vitamin therapy
and correction of the dietary deficiency.

The onset of senile dementia is insidious and some years may pass
before others note that the patient is commencing his dotage. Memory
defect is perhaps first noted by the patient. The defect is not so much in
immediate retention as in the rapid fading of impressions. Thus a
patient comes to see a physician. At the end of the interview she appears

---

[9] Ewalt, Strecker and Ebaugh. *Practical Clinical Psychiatry*, p. 149.

to be dazed. The physician says "You seem troubled." She answers "How am I going to get home?" The relatives are called on the phone and the physician is told that the patient came with the chauffeur in their car. Investigation showed that the chauffeur was quietly waiting to take her home.

Long before such an extreme defect of memory the patient may note that it is hard for him to acquire new information by reading. He understands perfectly, but does not retain. The synthetic sense is normal but there is a serious defect of memory. Then there may be a peculiar defect of consciousness—moments like a "petit mal" seizure in which the patient is dazed and does not see the relation of the moment just past to the present moment and does not know how to step into the immediate future. This may be due to a circulatory disturbance of some kind. Arteriosclerotic conditions often complicate senile dementia.

Naturally with extensive cortical destruction loss of emotional control results; and so some aged persons in whom one never noticed any show of impatience become irritable; and the good natured may become depressed. If however the patient has been well schooled in the importance of living up to all the virtues, sanctity may have risen to the therapeutic level and control may increase keeping pace with its own deterioration and grow like the incisors of rodents as fast as they are worn down by gnawing. As in other forms of mental disorder the *strength of the personality acquired in a holy life* may be a contributing factor to a peaceful old age, in which one looks forward with hope to the joys of eternal life. And yet should one who had lived a good and holy life become irritable in his old age we should not hold it against him for there are storms in which no skipper can save the boat.

4. Chronic Brain Syndrome Associated with Cerebral Arteriosclerosis

The mental picture in cerebral arteriosclerosis resembles that in senile dementia and in the terminal stages the two conditions are often indistinguishable. In both we have loss of emotional control and defects of interpretation, memory and judgment. But in arteriosclerotic conditions "spotted" gross defects of interpretation are more common. Thus visual agnosia (inability to interpret pictures) and sensory aphasia (inability to understand the spoken word) with other functions relatively intact are more common in arteriosclerosis. But we must remember that the two disorders are not always sharply differentiated, because purely senile changes due to wasting of tissues with age and microscopic to gross hemorrhages due to "breaking" of the hardened arteries (arteriosclerosis) may occur in one and the same patient. Memory defects in arteriosclerosis may involve the remote past and on the whole come on earlier than in senile dementia. In the senile condition the outstanding defect is the quick fading of memory for recent events and material that one tries to memorize.

But what distinguishes arteriosclerotic conditions from senile are two important symptoms: (a) the coming and going of sensory defects and similar fluctuations in memory and the power of emotional control, and (b) the sudden appearance of paralytic strokes involving muscles on one or both sides of the body.

Let us take the last illness of M. Louis Martin, the father of St. Thérèse of Lisieux as an example of "chronic brain syndrome associated with cerebral arteriosclerosis."

The account is based on *The Father of the Little Flower* by the Sister of St. Thérèse, Sister Genevieve of the Holy Face.[10] The work is replete with facts derived not merely from memory but also from letters of the period and entries in her personal diary.[11] Seeing that we have pointed out that the symptoms in the organic psychoses are determined not only by defects in the brain but by the prepsychotic character, it will be well to give an outline of the personality of Louis Martin.

5. The Personality of Louis Martin

M. Louis Martin was born August 22, 1823. He died July 29th, 1894. When about 20 he tried to enter the Religious Order of the Great St. Bernard (Alps). Deficiency in Latin blocked this ambition. He then learned watch making. In 1858 he married Zelie Guerin, having opened a watch and jewelry store at Alençon.

He was a vigorous martial personality. He was the son of a French army officer who for his service in war was decorated with the Cross of Knights of the Royal Military Order of St. Louis. M. Martin was a good swimmer and several times saved others from drowning. Personal danger meant nothing to him when anyone was in need. He was afraid of nothing.

---

[10] The Newman Press, Westminster Md., 1955. But see the psychiatrists's diagnosis reported in Stephane-Joseph Piat. *The Story of a Family*, New York, Kenedy, 1948, pp. 384-385. Footnote 1.

[11] Op. cit., p. 81.

His martial spirit and absolute fearlessness enabled him to do at times things that would have gotten others into trouble. "Once a local pilgrimage returning from Lourdes encountered in the station at Alencon a crowd which had come to jeer at them. Assuming the cause of the pilgrims he went to the head of the frightened group and, wearing a large carved wood rosary round his neck, he passed boldly through the midst of the crowd which stopped jeering and quickly dispersed."[12]

Father George Deshon, a member of the Paulist Fathers, was a West Point graduate and had known service in the United States Army. A mob was rioting near the Paulist Church. He went out and stood before them and told them in tones of West Point authority to disperse and go home. And strange to say they did. He and Louis Martin had what might be termed a vigorous military personality.

When we think of the martial elements in Louis Martin's character, it is readily seen that he would never allow his children to follow their own whims and depart from standards of righteous behavior and good etiquette that he wanted to establish. He loved each child with a most tender affection; and they loved him. But they learned to obey.

We might speak of Louis Martin as the soldier of Christ who always espoused the cause of anyone in need of help whenever and wherever he met him. He and his wife met a poor old tramp on the road: they brought him home, gave him a hearty meal, got better clothes and shoes for him, told him to come back whenever he was in want and finally arranged to have him accepted by the Little Sisters of the Poor.[13] His charity not merely gave a dime but espoused a cause.

His charity to others flowed from his life with God. Every morning he and his wife went to an early Mass. Every afternoon he made a visit to the Blessed Sacrament. He was a faithful member of the society of Nocturnal Adoration, arrived early and picked the most inconvenient hours for his period of adoration.

When at Alençon, "he purchased outside the town a small property called the Pavilion, with a hexagonal tower at the corner of the garden, where he used to retire to read quietly and to pray, having kept his taste for the life of the cloister."[14] When he moved to Lisieux,

---

[12]Op. cit., p. 9.
[13]Op. cit., p. 20.
[14]Op. cit., p. 3.

he made the third story of their home serve the same purpose and termed it the Belvedere.[15]

St. Thérèse of Lisieux may have imbibed her "little way" from the example of her father. He never made any comment on the things served him at table. "He would on no account suggest what things he liked best."[16] When asked why he did not smoke cigarettes he replied: "Must we not practice a little mortification?"[17] When he went on a journey he travelled third class to be assimilated to the poor.[18]

The way of little acts of self denial prepared him for the great sacrifice of giving all his five daughters to God in the religious life. Céline remained with him to the end; but he knew of her intention to enter Carmel.

He was very much pleased with a picture she painted for him and suggested that she study art in some Academy in Paris. She then told of her desire to enter Carmel. He wept with joy, and exclaimed with rapture:

"Come, Céline, let us go together before the Blessed Sacrament to thank the Lord for all the graces He has granted our family, and for the honor He had done me in choosing spouses in my home."[19]

About a year after his first attack of paralysis M. Martin paid a visit to his old parish church at Alencon. Three of his daughters were already in Carmel. He felt that he had done everything in his power for the holy children God had given him. He wanted to do more. Perhaps he felt that the heights of sanctity are infinite and he fain would lift his children to still higher levels. He had offered to God all that he had. He wanted to offer more. So he gave himself to God as a victim soul. On his return, he visited his three children in Carmel.

"Children, I have returned from Alençon, where I received in the Church of Notre Dame such signal graces and such consolations that I made this prayer: '*My God, it is too much! I am too happy; it is impossible to go to Heaven this way. I wish to suffer something for you, and I offered myself . . .*' The verb *victim* expired on his lips, writes Thérèse, he did not wish to pronounce it before us, but we understood."[20]

---

[15]Op. cit., p. 2.
[16]Op. cit., p. 27.
[17]Op. cit., p. 28.
[18]Op. cit., p. 29.
[19]Op. cit., p. 75.
[20]*The Father of the Little Flower* by the Sister of St. Thérèse. Newman Press, Westminster, Md., 1955, p. 84.

Let us now attempt an outline picture of the character of Louis Martin:

Perhaps the greatest light that comes to us on the character of any man is that which we receive through a knowledge of his ideals. From what we have written it seems clear that the guiding ideal of Louis Martin was to love God and do His work in the world. It was no empty dream. He lived with God a life of love and service. His morning presence at the Holy Sacrifice of the Mass, his afternoon visit to the Blessed Sacrament, his retirement at times during the day to the tower he had bought for that precise purpose when he lived at Alençon or its substitute, the third floor, the Belvedere, in his house at Lisieux, all these customs show us the center of his thoughts and the focus of his affections throughout his life.

The complement to the love, adoration and service of God is voluntary association with Christ in His Passion by a life of self-denial and suffering. This was true in an eminent degree of Mr. Martin.

Turning now to the more sensory side of his personality he was one who had himself in perfect emotional control. "Even on very moving occasions he did not allow himself to be excited, and remained perfectly the master of his feelings."[21]

We must recall in this summary his martial spirit, his great bravery in helping others in danger, his habit of responding to the needs of others, by making their cause his own, even at great inconvenience and expense to himself; and we see both from the spiritual and natural point of view a truly vigorous, worthwhile and holy personality.[22]

6. Mr. Martin's Last Illness

Mr. Martin's last illness hung on for about seven years. We may consider it as an illustration of chronic brain syndrome associated with cerebral arteriosclerosis. We have already pointed out that its two most characteristic symptoms are (a) fluctuations in the level of consciousness, memory and emotional control and (b) a series of paralytic strokes due to more or less extensive brain hemorrhages.

On May 1st 1887 Mr. Martin woke up and his entire left side was paralyzed. "He spoke rather inarticulately and dragged his leg."[23]

---

[21]Op. cit., p. 84.
[22]In these words the author does not wish to forestall the decision of the Church in the process of canonization now impending.
[23]The Father of the Little Flower, p. 83.

"Apart from some lapses of memory, he recovered sufficiently to take
an active interest in the confidences of Thérèse regarding her vocation,
and to accompany her in all its different steps. He had two other
paralytic strokes in the course of the year."[24] Towards the end of May
1888 "he began to show signs of more emotionalism and tears came
easily and frequently to his eyes.[25] This situation continued with
alternation of improvement and relapse."[26]

We have also pointed out that in mental disorders due to chronic
brain involvement the mental state is in part determined by the
patient's previous habits of thought. The following passage is a statement of fact not the imagination of an affectionate child: "Even when
confused, all the thoughts of our good father remained directed
towards God's service, which had been the center of his whole life, and
his acquired virtues continued to manifest themselves in spiritual
works of charity."[27]

He was well enough to be present on the clothing day of Thérèse,
January 10th 1889. But soon after "there were fresh lapses of memory
with new and stronger congestive strokes."[28] On February 12th of the
same year it was decided to take him to a mental home. He realized
the nature of the place as soon as he entered. There was no complaint,
only humility and surrender to Divine Providence. When Leonie and
Céline would go to visit him, he used to repeat constantly: "I am very
well here and I am here because it is the will of God. I needed this
trial. Besides I can do good around here. How many need conversion."[29]

Later he said to the doctor: "I was always accustomed to command,
and here I have to obey, it is hard! But I know why God has sent me
this trial. I never had any humiliation in my life: I needed one."
The doctor replied: "Well! This one can count."

He continued his little acts of self-denial and would not eat cake in
Holy Week. When well enough he went daily to Mass and received
Holy Communion.

In May 1892 his legs were completely paralyzed. He was brought

[24]Loc cit.
[25]P. 84.
[26]P. 86.
[27]P. 86.
[28]P. 91.
[29]P. 92.

back to Lisieux and on the 12th taken to see his daughters in Carmel. On June the 29th 1894, Céline was watching by his bed all alone. He seemed unconscious then opened his eyes on Céline, gazed on her with affection and inexpressible gratitude. Then closed them for ever.[30]

The last illness of Louis Martin is not only an illustration of the development of mental symptoms in arteriosclerosis but also a beautiful picture of sanctity at its therapeutic level: "It is remarkable that even in his attacks of nervousness or of sadness, he never showed signs of revolt nor of any violent or unbecoming behavior."[31] The beautiful normal personality of Louis Martin did not deteriorate with the impairment of his brain by arteriosclerosis, but was maintained till he closed his eyes in death.

Thus did great holiness show its power to maintain the vigor of the personality in spite of ever increasing damage to the brain.

---

[30]P. 114.
[31]P. 103.

III. Nature and Grace in the Making of a Saint

CHAPTER XIX

The True Light That Enlightens Every Man

1. Man and His Brute Instincts

Is there any way in which the human mind is enlightened and led on by God Himself toward the Eternal Good? Or is man blind to the Eternal Good and able only to experience a driving power to action that comes from his lower animal nature masked in the depths of the unconscious? An affirmative answer to the first question is fundamental Catholic doctrine. Father Robo denies the first question and affirms the second in the following words:

"In the dim recesses of the unconscious lurk in us all some innate inclinations, unreasoned instincts. Allotted to each one in uneven proportions, they are the basic elements of our characters. Some of them are called bad, not because they are so in themselves, but because they are so powerful that we easily lose control of them. They seem to have their roots in a life force, the will to exist and to exist in the fullest possible manner. They are the driving power behind all human activities, and lacking it we should lead the inert life of the sloth on his tree. Without ambition, who would assume the burdens of government? Would trade or industry flourish if no one cared for money? Should we trouble to cook and to eat, if we took no pleasure in our food? Would a bare sense of duty be strong enough to induce men to raise a family?"[1]

There can be no doubt about the existence and power of animal drives in human beings. But because man is an animal, must we deny that he is rational? Because there are selfish politicians who seek only themselves, must we deny the existence of true statesmen whose conduct is motivated dominantly by a genuine love for the fatherland?

---

[1] Rev. Etienne Robo, *The Two Portraits*, 2nd Ed. Newman Press, Westminster, Md., 1957, pp. 78-79.

Do any work in the light of the noble ideals they have honestly worked out for the welfare of their fellow citizens? Were all those who signed the Declaration of Independence seeking selfish personal ambitions and not the true good of the thirteen colonies? Do all men live merely to eat, or is it possible for some to live for the higher things in life: religion, science, art, music, poetry? Are all marriages based solely on sex craving or can some truly see in the establishment of a home that will be a school of the service of God a duty and a joy that transcends all other considerations?

2. God's Law in the Mind of Man

Let us consider the problem from the point of view of the concept of God recognized by the Church. God is Infinite Intelligence and Almighty Power. His very essence is the Eternal Law according to which all things were given the nature of their being and by which they are directed to the ends for which they were created.

The nonliving world is directed by God: The Eternal Law: by inexorable laws of nature from which they cannot depart. These same laws operate in the plant world and throughout all nature; but there resides in every germ a new type of activity a formal cause by which each germ organizes a living organism true to its type. In the world of animals still other laws are recognized: "innate inclinations, unreasoned instincts," to use the words of Father Robo, by which, under the guidance of sensory percepts, they grow, develop and fill their place in nature and scintillate the brightness of their Creator.

As St. Thomas says: "Law is nothing else than a rule of practical reason in the mind of the person in supreme authority who governs any complete social unit. Granted the truth that Divine Providence rules the world, it is evident that the entire cosmos is governed by Divine Reason. Therefore the very concept, of the government of things, existing in God, the Supreme Authority, in the cosmos, has in itself the essence of *law*. Since, therefore, in the Divine Mind concepts do not come and go with time, but the Divine Concept is eternal, as is said in the Book of Proverbs,[2] it follows that the Law of God (governing all things) should be called *Eternal*."[3]

---

[2] The reference is to the whole beautiful chapter eight of the Book of Proverbs recounting God's action in establishing the universe in all its parts in which we read "I (Wisdom) was set up from eternity and of old before the earth was made." (verse 23).

[3] Summa Theologica, 1.2. Q. XCI, i, corpus.

When now we consider man in the light of the Eternal Law we see that he differs from the brute creation whose nature cannot rise above unreasoned instincts. Brute animals feel the force of the law that governs them but they cannot know either the law or the Lawgiver. But man can and does know the moral law by which he is governed and the Eternal Wisdom by Whom he is bound by the law of right conduct. "That which is known of God is manifest in them (the Gentiles). For God hath manifested it unto them. For the invisible things of Him from the creation of the world are clearly seen, being understood by the things that are made. His eternal power also and divinity: so that they are inexcusable." (Romans I:19-20). *God therefore makes Himself known naturally to the human mind.*

But God also expresses in the human mind a knowledge of the Eternal Law in so far as it *directs the mind of man to know and serve Him: the Eternal Good.* "For when the Gentiles, who have not the law, do by nature those.things that are of the law: these having not the law, are a law to themselves. Who shew the work of the law written in their hearts their conscience bearing witness to them." (Romans II:14-15).

The Eternal Law written in the mind of man is termed the *Natural Law*. It is fundamentally the same in all races of mankind.

It is reasonable that the Eternal Wisdom Who "reacheth from end to end mightily and ordereth all things sweetly" (Wisdom VIII:1) should not only make known Himself to the minds of man, and write the law in their hearts that they must obey, but also implant in every rational creature a natural inclination to that which is consonant with the Eternal Law.[4] True, this natural inclination may be weakened by vice, but it can also be strengthened by virtue. When it is strengthened by virtue it can become stronger than any animal drive and men "do by nature those things that are of the law" and "having not the law are a law to themselves" and "show the work of the law written in their hearts."

This inclination to observe the Natural Law which God has written in the heart of man, a law that only an intelligent being is capable of understanding, cannot be termed an "unreasoned instinct," nor can it be said that "innate inclinations," unreasoned instincts constitute "the driving force behind all human activities and lacking it we should lead the inert life of the sloth on his tree." This fundamentally

---

[4] St. Thomas S.T. 1.2., Q.XCIII, vi, corpus.

Freudian doctrine is incompatible with Holy Scripture. It cannot be applied even to pagans before the coming of Christ. It is contrary to the teaching of the Church on grace and free will. For there can be no free will if man can act only in response to innate unreasoning instincts masked in the unconscious.

3. Divine Helps that Transcend Nature

God's illumination of the human mind by the natural law, and the inclination of his will to obey, is natural and not supernatural. It does not pertain to the order of grace and would exist in what is termed the *state of pure nature*. But *homo sapiens* has ever existed in a state in which he has been called to a supernatural end: to know God and see Him as He is and live in love for Him in eternity.

Consequently, even before a man is endowed with sanctifying grace and elevated to a supernatural state, man received from time to time over and above the light of the natural law and a natural inclination to observe it, special supernatural illuminations of his intellect and inspirations of his will through which he learns about his supernatural end and yearns to attain it.

The following example will explain what is here meant by the illumination of grace:

A lawyer in a western town had watched for some time a little old woman, a widow, who supported her children by doing housework. We are not told whether the lawyer belonged to some church or was without any religion. But morning after morning he always saw the little old woman making her way up a steep hill to the Catholic Church. One icy morning he had great difficulty in battling his way to the office over streets covered with sheets of sleet. He made a bet with himself that the little old woman would not be climbing the hill to the Church that day.

"When he looked out, his heart rose in his throat. As he said many times afterward: 'Tears came to my eyes as I watched. There was the old dear on her hands and knees crawling up that icy hill.'

He was so affected that he closed his office and went home. He burst into the house and terrified the young Irish servant girl by shouting at her: 'Are you a Catholic?' She was so frightened at the unexpected question and the disruption of the usually smooth-running house that all she could do was nod. 'Do you have any books about it?' Again she nodded. My grandfather continued: 'Please go get them.

I want to see what it is in that Church that makes a woman crawl up a hill on her hands and knees to get to it.' "[5]

The result of his study was the conversion of himself and all his family.

Let us look at certain elements in this account. It starts with seeing an old woman climbing up a steep hill over the ice covered streets in order to get to church. This incident is an example of what is often termed an *external* grace. But theologians tell us that though such external events are sometimes called graces, in a loose sense of the word "grace," the term grace is properly used only of the interior illumination by God of the intellect and the inner inspiration of the will.[6] Furthermore this illumination of the intellect and inspiration of the will to be a true grace must evidently be produced by God and not the natural effect of the workings of the mind.

We also note an emotional condition in the lawyer manifested by tears and a profound disturbance of his ordinary stable mental equilibrium, associated with a drive to investigate the teachings of the Catholic Church. The emotional elements in the situation are also often termed graces in a loose sense of the word. Such activities of our lower nature as feelings, emotions, sensory desires and fears often transpire in a process of conversion and they seem to be used by God directly or indirectly in the more or less long drawn out process of the conversion of a soul to the faith or to the leading of a perfect spiritual life. "We are not accustomed to call these internal movements of the sensory faculties graces. In the *strict theological sense* an interior salutary grace is understood to be something bestowed on the higher, that is, spiritual, faculties, for only these faculties, namely intellect and will, are capable of eliciting truly supernatural acts."[7]

But the lawyer received a truly intellectual illumination: "There is something beyond all my past experience in the sacrifice of the 'old dear on her hands and knees crawling up that icy hill.' " Her religion may truly come from God. And then there was a strong impulse given to his will. "I must investigate her religion at once."

---

[5] *The Way to Emmaus*. Ed. by John A. O'Brien, New York, McGraw-Hill, 1953, p. 206-207.

[6] Ad. Tanquery, *Synopsis Theologiae Dogmaticae*, New York, Benziger, 24th Ed., 1938, Vol. 3, pp. 103-104.

[7] Ludovicus Lercher, S. J., *Institutiones Theologicae Dogmaticae*, 4th Ed., Herder, Barcelona, 1945, Vol. IV, 1, p. 2620.

Evidently the lawyer was not following the drive of innate inclinations and unreasoning instincts rising from the dim recesses of the unconscious. Unreasoning instincts can, as Father Robo points out, seek food and sex satisfaction; but they know nothing of God and religion. What made the lawyer close his office and go home and seek at once information about the Catholic Church, was a new conscious intellectual idea that arose in his mind and a new drive, never known before, to get information about the Catholic Church. The profound effect upon his mind, the intensity of his drive to know the Church came from nothing innate, and nothing in all his past experience. God used the example of an old woman to illumine his mind and inspire his will.

CHAPTER XX

The Higher Criticism in Hagiography

CAN A TRUER picture of a saint be obtained by applying to the data of his life the technique of psychoanalysis?

Heretofore we have had two types of biographies in hagiography.

1. An older type such as we find in *The Golden Legend of Jacobus de Voragine*,[1] a work written in the thirteenth century to edify.

2. A more modern type based upon painstaking historical research in which one tries to present the picture of the saint as he was in life by a study of the state of society in his day, actual examples of his conduct, passages from his letters, an analysis of his thought as revealed in his writings.

A recent book[2] by Father Robo suggests the possibility of a new departure in hagiography and so we would have:

3. The psychoanalytic picture of a saint.

The new method in hagiography, as used by Father Robo, raises a problem: Can the true picture of a saint be drawn when one eliminates everything of a supernatural character in his life and in the motivation of his conduct?

There will be two answers to this question. The true Freudians will say: Most certainly, for all religion is a delusion. We must therefore eliminate what is apparently supernatural in order to get the true picture of a saint.

But the theist will say: We must pause and make first a critical study of psychoanalytic methods before we undertake this task. But this all important preliminary is lacking in Father Robo's book. He makes no attempt at a critical evaluation of his technique, which bears a close resemblance to psychoanalytic method and theory. He gives no

---

[1] Translated and adapted from the Latin by Granger Ryan and Helmut Ripperger, New York, Longmans, 1948.

[2] Etienne Robo, *Two Portraits of St. Thérèse of Lisieux*, Chicago, Regnery, 1955, 2nd Ed. Westminster, Md., Newman, 1957.

discussion nor history of his technique which is based on the "mental mechanism" of "rationalization." He does not discuss its limitations nor the principles on which it was founded in the past nor his acceptance, modification or rejection of those principles. But without such a discussion we cannot properly estimate the work he has laid before the public. Let us first say something on the concept of rationalization and the study of character.

1. Rationalization and the Study of Character

Perhaps the "source concept" for the understanding of rationalization is Freud's theory of human impulses.

All impulses derive, according to Freud, from a stimulation or irritation of some organ of the body. The aim of the impulse is to eliminate this stimulus or irritation. But every organ gives rise to two different forms of excitement. Freud writes as follows:

"Another preliminary assumption in the theory of the impulse which we cannot relinquish, states that the bodily organs furnish two kinds of excitement which are determined by differences of a chemical nature. One of these forms of excitement we designate as the specifically sexual, and the concerned organ as the *erogenous zone,* while the sexual element emanating from it is the partial impulse."[3] It thus appears that in all drives to action there must be always a sexual component, according to Freud. He conceives of this sexual component entering into all movements toward higher cultural accomplishments. Their driving force is in reality the seeking of sexual satisfaction under the cloak of the betterment of mankind. When one interprets his own conduct by high moral or religious ideals he is *rationalizing.* If we analyze his behavior we shall uncover the true though unconscious springs of his action: ultimately the satisfaction of sexual desire.

Father Robo holds a similar concept and expresses it as follows:

"In the dim recesses of the unconscious lurk in us all some innate inclinations, unreasoned instincts. Allotted to each one in uneven proportions, they are the basic elements of our characters. Some of them are called bad, not because they are so in themselves, but because they are so powerful that we easily lose control of them. They seem to have their roots in a life force, the will to exist and to exist in the fullest possible manner. They are the driving power behind all

---

[3] *Three Contributions to Sexual Theory*, transl. by Brill, 1916, p. 33.

HEROIC SANCTITY AND INSANITY

human activities, and lacking it we should lead the inert life of the sloth on his tree."[4]

"We are not disparaging St. Teresa when we assert that she was naturally proud, self-willed and obstinate. It only means that she was a daughter of Adam, and that, because she was a saint, she fought and conquered these inclinations."[5] There is no objection to calling a saint a child of Adam. But there is very serious objection to saying that the children of Adam have only one driving power in all their activities and that this derives from "innate inclinations, unreasoned instincts." If this is so there is no essential difference between the children of Adam and the children of brute animals.

Catholic philosophy recognizes two different driving forces in human nature: one derives from what can be perceived by the senses and the other from that which can be perceived by the intellect. Each gives rise to what St. Thomas termed an *appetitus*. In using this term he was following Cicero who also distinguished between impulsive and rational desires.[6] "There are two kinds of desires: a sensory, namely, and an intellectual which is termed will . . . The object of each is the good, but different kinds of good. The object of sensory desire is a good apprehended by sense. But the object of intellectual desire or the will is the good under its general aspect as it can be apprehended by the intellect. The object of charity is no sensory good but the divine good which is known by the intellect alone."[7] Father Robo makes divine charity something that has no warmth. "Can any woman, he asks, be entirely satisfied with a love of reason and will?"[8]

But we must never forget that the perception of the Divine Good leads us where no sensory desire could conduct. It is truly a genuine driving force of human nature without which human activity cannot be explained. The principle of Father Robo that we should all be inactive like a sloth in a tree were it not for our sensory "innate inclinations, unreasoned instincts" is a fundamental error. It is a strongly Freudian-toned theory. What was the source of the enthusiasm of St. Francis Xavier on his missions? Freud would answer cloaked sensuality.

---

[4] *The Two Portraits*, p. 64, 2nd Ed. pp. 78-79.
[5] Op. cit., p. 65, 2nd Ed. p. 79.
[6] See quotation in Harper's Latin Dictionary. Cic. Off. 1, 28, 101.
[7] *Summa Theologica*, 2.2. Q. XXIV, 1, corpus.
[8] *The Two Portraits*, p. 137. See above p. 70 on the bodily resonance of intellectual realizations: love of God and sorrow for sin.

Father Robo's answer is cloaked innate inclinations, unreasoned instincts.

St. Thérèse, as we shall see, attributed the beginning of her Carmelite vocation to the example of her sister Pauline. But she tells us that there came a time when she "wanted to enter Carmel, not for Pauline, but for Jesus only." (See below p. 195). In other words her one dominant reason was the love of God. But Father Robo cannot admit this for "the one driving force behind all human activities consists in innate inclinations, unreasoned instincts. She did not truly want to go to Carmel because of her love for Christ, but out of pride, self-will, and obstinacy. This concept is theologically unsound because it *cannot be reconciled with the Church's teaching on grace*. The illumination of the mind and inspiration of the will by the Holy Spirit are necessary in the sanctification of the soul, along with man's cooperation.[9] But innate inclinations, unreasoned instincts are incapable of leading man to the ideals of sanctity.

Father Robo's principle that these innate sensory instinctive drives are the driving power behind all human activities is *incompatible with Catholic philosophy*. Only that which is in some manner perceived can lead to desire and give rise to a drive to action. Sense cannot perceive the things of the spirit. Consequently, the activities of the spiritual life can never be explained on the basis of "innate unreasoned instincts."

Our Holy Father Pius XII, while granting that it is possible to use the methods of psychoanalysis without prejudice to religion, seems to have rejected the pansexualism of Freud.[10] On the other hand, Freud's concept of two forms of excitement, one specific to the organ the other sexual emanating from every organ of the body, has no solid foundation in biology; and is rejected by many, if not most, psychiatrists of today.[11] With Freud there is also no such thing as ideals

---

[9] Council of Trent, Denzinger-Bannwart, 797, 813, 814.

[10] "It is not proved—it is in fact, incorrect—that the pansexual method of a certain school of psychoanalysis is an indispensable integrating part of all psychotherapy which is serious and worthy of the name." Trans. of an article in L'osservatore Romano of Sept. 21, 1952, Interpreting the Address of His Holiness Pius XII. Pamphlet. Natl. Catholic Welfare Conference. *The Moral Limits of Medical Research and Treatment*. An Address of Pius XII, September 14, 1952, p. 12.

[11] Eugene Kahn, Professor of Psychiatry at Yale, speaks of the repudiation by the clinician "of the pansexualism of the Freudian teaching" *Psychopathic Personalities*, New Haven, Yale Univ. Press. 1931, p. 3.

and motives being instilled into the mind by God for the very concepts of God and religion are delusions.

2. Rationalization in Daily Life

There is no question but that rationalization is a "mental mechanism" a spontaneous trend, in many situations in daily life. Take for example any young priest commencing his work for souls. He loves to preach because of the opportunity it gives him to turn the minds and hearts of the people to God. And in so thinking he is perfectly honest and true. He notices his reputation growing and takes genuine delight in the fact. The idea comes to him the real reason I love to preach is that it tickles my vanity. I want to be praised by men. Should he, therefore, give up preaching because it tickles his vanity? This is not allowed him because it is his duty to preach. So he settles down to the fact that there are two reasons why he wants to preach (a) to turn souls to God; (b) to increase his good reputation. If he wants to arrive at a true estimate of the relative power of his motives, let him ask himself would I stop preaching even if no one ever said to me, "O Father, what a lovely sermon?" I think practically every good preacher could say honestly to himself even though I received mockery instead of praise, I would go on doing my duty and preach the word of God.

In other words, in using "the technique of rationalization" one must realize that it does not lead to a complete disjunction of motives: either those that come from high moral and spiritual ideals or those that come from low and unworthy selfishness. The cockle and the wheat ordinarily grow together in the same mind until the day of judgment. But *as sanctity increases the wheat crowds out the cockle.* We might say that if a soul has attained to the heroic practice of virtue we should suspect any argument that concludes to the presence of active selfishness playing a significant role in, much less dominating, the life of a heroic soul.

St. Augustine, looking back over his life, shows us how he recognized that "rationalization" had played a part in his own life. It is quite likely that even at the time he wrote his confessions the selfishness he detected in the past was already dead. He remembered how praises had been showered upon him. But he thought of the good that would come to the Church because of the existence in it of prelates worthy of praise. And thought to himself that he *could* therefore be glad because he was praised. In our language of today, he thought of this as a piece of rationalization and wrote thus of how he detected it: "Behold in Thee, O Truth, I see that I ought not to be moved at my own praises, for my own sake, but for the good of my neighbor. And whether it be so with me, I know not. For herein I know less of myself than of Thee. I beseech now, O my God, discover to me myself also, that I may confess unto my brethren, who are to pray for me, wherein I find myself maimed. Let me examine myself again more diligently. If in my praise I am moved with the good of my neighbor, why am I less moved if another be unjustly dispraised than if it be myself?" We see then how a great saint can be deceived by "rationalization" and also how by prayer and self-analysis he lays bare his error.

3. Analysis of Character by "the Technique of Rationalization"
    With the Freudians the analysis of character by the technique of rationalization assumes their fundamental principle: the ultimate motivation of conduct is always in its essence a sexual drive. Father Robo does not lay down this principle, nor does he analyze his technique so as to give expression to any principle. But as we shall see from certain examples, that we shall study later, the conclusions he reaches demand for their validity the assumption that if a selfish motive may be conceived of as dominating conduct, the higher moral and religious motives to which St. Thérèse may attribute her conduct are products of rationalization and not the real determining factors in what she does.
    When a Freudian analyst has a patient before him he attempts to analyze the real motives of a patient's behavior (in the light of Freudian pansexualism) by the analysis of dreams and the spontaneous flow of thought of the patient during the analysis (free association). By the associations thus at his disposal he endeavors to lead the patient to see the sexual motivation of his behavior and one might say pushes the analysis till this end is accomplished. When, however, the patient is dead and one has the writings he left behind, the task is much more difficult. Without careful and constant precautions and some kind of checking with all available biographical material the analyst may present a fiction of his own and not the character of the person he is studying.
    I remember listening to a paper read at St. Elizabeth's Hospital, Washington, D.C.—early, I think, in 1918. Psychiatrists were there from various parts of the country for training in the understanding of

the "mental mechanisms" of behavior. Dr. William A. White, an outstanding figure in American psychiatry was presiding and a distinguished member of the staff read the paper. It was a psychoanalysis of Charles Darwin. The fact that Darwin wrote a paper on the fertilization of orchids, demonstrated, to the essayist, that he suffered from abnormal sexual curiosity. His interest in animals was taken as evidence of bestiality. Something else proved homosexuality and the final conclusion was that Darwin was a polymorphous sexual pervert. When the paper concluded Dr. White asked for criticisms. No one rose to criticize or ask a question. As it were in despair Dr. White turned to me and said: "Father Moore, won't you please say something about this paper." Seeing that the paper raised the whole question of the Freudian technique in the analysis of character I rose and developed the following points: The essayist has taken the work of Charles Darwin as the dream of his life. He has analyzed this "dream" as any psychoanalyst analyzes the dream of a patient by getting associations with words and phrases in the dream; but with this difference: He did not have the associations of Charles Darwin. When we take a dream of one patient and present it to another patient we do not get the associations of the dreamer, but of one who has heard the dream without having dreamt it. And so what we get is not what the dream meant to the dreamer, but what it meant to this other person.[12] Whose associations has Dr. ———— made use of? Not Darwin's, but his own. He has, therefore, analyzed not Darwin, but himself.

The technique of dream analysis, by itself without recourse to an author's biography, cannot be used in the interpretation of a dead author's writings. But they are the products of his mind and often the expression of his ideals. If we take an author's works *in conjunction* with his letters and the data of biographers who knew him personally we can often add something from the interior life of a poet or novelist to the account of the biographer.

Now it is something of that kind that Father Robo has attempted. But when we examine the matter carefully we see that Father Robo has in his own mind, generalized the fundamental Freudian principle: The ultimate driving force of human nature is always sexual. With Father Robo the principle becomes: The ultimate driving force of

---

[12] A psychiatrist who works with group therapy told me he has often demonstrated this to be true by having the whole group write down their associations to the words and phrases of the dream of one member of the group.

human nature is not of a moral and spiritual nature but some form of self-seeking. As our essayist used his own associations with the words and phrases in the works of Charles Darwin, Father Robo takes some selfish motive that comes to his mind and makes that the true motive in the conduct of St. Thérèse. The high moral and spiritual motives, that she may allege, he takes as indicating mere rationalizations[13] by which she blinds herself to the real motives of her conduct. One might say that this is his general technique of procedure, not a rare exception, but the rule.

Strange to say he makes no room in the picture he discusses of St. Thérèse for the direction of her thought and conduct by ideals and impulses that are in their essence illuminations of the mind and inspirations of the will caused by divine grace. "We are not trying to apportion the respective shares of grace and of nature in the attitude of Thérèse towards others. We only register her sayings and actions as we find them in the autobiography."[14] That may be. But can you give a true picture of the mind of a canonized saint—whom Holy Mother Church, by her canonization, has decided has attained to the heroic practice of virtue—without introducing into the picture of her character the ideals and impulses that came from God and led her on to the practice of heroic virtue?

A well known Dominican theologican answered our questions, as follows, long before the appearance of *The Two Portraits*.

"One demands of a physician trained in psychiatry that he should know psychiatry when he speaks to us of his patients, without supposing that he should be required to be a theologian to discuss God's workings in the souls of the saints. Nevertheless, one cannot explain sanctity without grace, nor the progress of the soul on its way toward perfection without a deep knowledge of Christian virtues and of the gifts of the Holy Spirit."[15] "A saint is an incarnation of the Gospel and of the highest principles of Christian spirituality."[16]

If one will study carefully *The Two Portraits* he will find only passing

---

[13]Father Robo never uses the word *rationalization*. But his interpretation of selfishness as the true motive of conduct in St. Thérèse implies what psychiatrists speak of as rationalization.
[14]Op. cit., 2nd Ed. p. 111.
[15]M. M. Philipon, Maître de Théologie, *Sainte Thérèse de Lisieux*. 3rd Ed. Desclee, 1946, pp. 8-9.
[16]Op. cit., p. 10.

references to anything like grace. Thus he writes of Thérèse at four: "Even at this tender age, her religion was the principal influence in her life and the mainspring of her actions."[17] One wonders if this is a slip of the pen when he had forgotten about the "unreasoned instincts that lurk in the dim recesses of the unconscious and are the driving power behind all human activities.[18] But he quickly passes from this slip of the pen to speak of another component in her character: her "astonishing will power which twelve or thirteen years later will make possible that undeviating, indomitable pursuit of perfection, which continued steadily for nine years and is perhaps the most remarkable feat of her holiness. If Christ said "without Me you can do nothing" (John XV:5) is it good theology to say without qualification that will power makes sanctity possible?

Heroic virtue means that grace is dominant in the soul and nature has retired into the background. Any attempt therefore to retire grace into the background and interpret conduct as a low form of natural selfishness gives a false picture of heroic virtue and betrays a naturalism incompatible with the ideals of the Church.

I may perhaps illustrate here what I mean by a comparison. One trained in the modern school of art was once asked to make a copy of an anatomical drawing of the outer, middle and inner ear. He knew nothing about the nature of what he was drawing except that the pinna of the external ear looked familiar. This was drawn so that it could be recognized. But a long black shadow (reaching down into the Eustachian tube) dominated the whole picture and made it hard to interpret. So Father Robo has made shadows dominate the picture of St. Thérèse's character. Not content with that, he has introduced shadows where none exist.

---

[17] *The Two Portraits*, 2nd Ed., p. 65.
[18] P. 79, 2nd Ed.

CHAPTER XXI

The Vocation of St. Thérèse

Is IT REALLY true that in discussing the spiritual life of St. Thérèse *The Two Portraits* retire grace into the background and interpret the conduct of St. Thérèse as a low form of natural selfishness? And, if so, is Father Robo in doing this merely acting as an impartial historian and, as he says of himself in the introduction, is merely "the servant of the evidence"?

Father Robo's account of the vocation of St. Thérèse is an example of his technique of "rationalization" in the interpretation of conduct. His account of her vocation follows immediately on his enunciation of the principle of "unreasoned instinct" in the unconscious as the driving power behind all human activities.

1. Father Robo's Account of the Vocation of St. Thérèse

He commences by explaining the technique of "rationalization." He does not use the word rationalization, but as we have explained above, this word is used by psychiatrists to describe the "mental mechanism" that Father Robo attributes to St. Thérèse in working out her vocation.

"She did not reach perfection all at once, and we must not be misled by her assurance that 'she had never done her own will.' That she was convinced of it goes without saying, for she was completely sincere, but, like many self-willed people, when she wanted something badly, and had made up her mind, she managed *always* to persuade herself that it was also the will of God. This is not particularly uncommon among superiors, and we ourselves have been informed sometimes by wilful people that they were obeying God's will, when they were only having their own way."[1]

The attractive element in this argument is the fact that sometimes

---

[1] Op. cit., 2nd Ed., p. 81.

people do "rationalize" in exactly this way.[2] The fallacy lies in the suggestion that no one can ever act on the basis of truly good motives in response to noble ideals. With Freud all motivation is necessarily sexual; and with Father Robo, unreasoning selfish drives welling up from the unconscious.

We have italicized the word *always* in the above quotation in order to raise the question whether or not Father Robo in this matter is as he claims only the servant of the evidence. A child who at the age of four commenced to count her little sacrifices must have, on many occasions, wanted many things badly and have given up her own will in order to do the will of God. Take for instance the incident when her Father had made arrangements for her and Céline to learn painting. On Thérèse's tenth birthday he called in the two, and having arranged the matter first with Céline the elder, he turned to Thérèse: " 'Well, little Queen, would you like to learn painting too?' I was going to say: 'Yes, indeed, I should' when Marie remarked that I had not the same taste for it as Céline. She carried her point and I said nothing, thinking it was a splendid opportunity to make a big sacrifice to Our Lord: I was so anxious to learn, that even now I wonder how I was able to keep silence."[3] For a child of ten this was an heroic sacrifice. She made it, "when she wanted something badly," for the love of God to gain grace for men.

Here Father Robo is not the servant of the evidence but has falsified the record. One might say from the time Thérèse was four years of age she schooled herself in giving up the things "she wanted badly" without an attempt to persuade herself that God wanted her to enjoy them.

Father Robo has merely modified the pansexualism of Freud and made selfishness rather than sexuality the one driving force in the life of St. Thérèse. Far from being a servant of the evidence he follows theory blindly without regard to the evidence. "If we have any doubts left," writes Father Robo, "about this young girl being as the novelist puts it 'wilful and obstinate to a prodigious degree' we need only observe the inflexible tenacity that took her to Bayeux and to Rome in pursuit of her plans. She had made up her mind that she must enter Carmel as a postulant . . . before the completion of her

---

[2] See T. V. Moore, *Cognitive Psychology*, Lippincott, Philadelphia, 1939, 394 ff.
[3] *Thérèse of Lisieux*, Trans. by T. N. Taylor, New York, Kenedy, 1924, p. 127, note.

fifteenth year."[4] He pictures St. Thérèse as going against the advice of everyone in her persistent drive to enter Carmel at fifteen. "She expresses her disappointment by floods of tears each time she is given some advice by the Superior, her uncle, her sister Marie, the Bishop, the Vicar General, and even by the Pope. She disagrees with them all because she alone knows the will of God, while the others are blind to it."[5] In these statements is Father Robo "attributing motives" without warrant or is he the servant of the evidence? Let us see.

2. St. Thérèse's Account of Her Vocation to Carmel

St. Thérèse traces the origin of her vocation to an incident that took place when she was about two years of age. "Sometimes I heard people saying that Pauline would be a nun, and, without quite knowing what it meant, I thought: 'I will be a nun too.' This is one of my first recollections and I have never changed my mind; so it was the example of this beloved sister which from the age of two, drew me to the Divine Spouse of Virgins."[6]

We may now ask the question whether or not this thought: "I will be a nun too" was the response of a child to a divine vocation. There would be no possibility of proving that it was to one who, like Freud, did not believe in the existence of God; nor to one who though he admitted the existence of God did not conceive of Him as the true light that enlighteneth every man who comes into this world. But one who believes that God directs the whole universe in its course and that God's dealings with men are intimated to us by Christ in the words: not a sparrow "shall fall on the ground without your Father" (Matthew X:29) and "better are you than many sparrows" (Matthew X:31), it is natural to think that the example of Pauline *might* have been God's first call to St. Thérèse to a religious life.

When we consider St. Thérèse's words: "This is one of my first recollections and I have never changed my mind" the evidence becomes very strong that Pauline's example was God's call to Thérèse. The mere whims of childhood come and go—the voice of God resounds forever.

Pauline's own vocation to Carmel has on it the stamp of God's

---

[4] Op. cit., p. 82.
[5] Op. cit., p. 71.
[6] *Soeur Thérèse of Lisieux, The Little Flower of Jesus.* Trans. by T. N. Taylor, New York, Kenedy. Ninth Impression 1924, p. 22, Manuscript page 6, right.

illuminating and inspiring grace. She wanted at the age of 20 to enter the Visitation convent of Le Mans. They told her to wait for three years. One morning the following incident took place which she described as follows: "I was present at the six o'clock Mass at St. Jacques in the chapel of Our Lady of Mt. Carmel. Suddenly my soul was filled with light and God showed me that it was not the Visitation that He wished me to enter, but Carmel. I had never considered Carmel before, and there I was possessed, in an instant, by an irresistible attraction towards it."[7]

We may look upon it as the general teaching of the Church that a true religious vocation is a special call from God.*

If a true religious vocation is a call from God it must be an illuminating and inspiring grace. But this does not mean that a religious vocation necessarily implies some kind of "interior locution."

---

[7] Quoted from Rev. F. Horsfield. *The Saint of Lisieux* "Pauline" July 1952, *5*, No. 3, p. 51.

*"Canon Lahitton in 1909 published a book *La vocation Sacerdotal*, Paris, 1909. This was followed by another *Deux conceptions divergentes de la vocation sacerdotal*, Paris, 1910. This gave rise to a controversy on the concept of a priestly vocation which he presented and the necessity in such a vocation of a conscious supernatural inclination of the mind. The matter having been presented to the Holy See, Pius X referred it to a special commission of Cardinals on June 20, 1912." (Joseph de Guibert, S. J. Documenta Ecclesiastica Christianae Perfectionis studium spectantia. Rome, Gregorian University, 1931, 612, p. 411.)

Canons 1353 and 1357 of Codex of Canon law speak of the "vocation" to the priesthood and seem to be at variance with the decree of this commission (AAS, t *4*, 485). Guibert says the wording of the decree seems to exclude any "interior call", whereas it merely excludes the necessity of such a call or a right to ordination arising from it. One might say that the decree does not take up the nature of the "call from God", but points out that a practical judgment on fitness for ordination must be based on evidence of a right intention and endowment by nature, grace, and training that give hope that the candidate will carry out well his priestly duties. Both forms of the twofold formula of the Society of Jesus approved by Julius III, Bulla, *Exposcit debitum*, July 21, 1550 speak of whether or not the Holy Spirit, Who impels the candidates for the Society, gives them enough grace to carry out their vocation (Guibert, op. cit., 358, p. 202).

St. Alphonsus in his Moral Theology, IV, Cap. 1, 78, raises the question: *Whether or not and to what extent anyone called by God to the religious life sins if he neglects to follow his vocation.* His answer is that *abstractly* it is no sin, because counsels do not oblige under pain of sin, but *concretely*, considering the danger into which he would precipitate himself, he would place his eternal salvation in grave danger. Pius XII termed the divine call the foundation of every vocation. A. A. S. May 31, 1956.

In general it is a silent wordless attraction. It may not be accompanied by a *certainty* that God is calling.

When St. Thérèse was about 9 years of age she "heard Pauline talking to Marie about soon entering Carmel."[8] She tells us of the anguish she felt from that time on realizing that Pauline was lost to her. Pauline tried to console her by explaining the religious life. "Then one evening, when I was thinking over the picture she had drawn, I felt that the Carmel was the desert where God wished me also to hide. I felt this so strongly that I had not the least doubt of it; nor was it a childish dream, but the certainty of a Divine Call. *I wanted to enter Carmel, not for Pauline, but for Jesus only.* This impression, which I cannot properly describe, left me with a feeling of inward peace."[9]

We might remark here that clearing the mind of doubts and leaving it in great inward peace is characteristic of a call that comes from God. It is usually accompanied by a strong impulse to ask advice about the matter; and, if encouraged, to do everything possible to obey the call.

3. Divine Calls and Pathological Stubbornness

Anyone with experience in the "history of vocations" will remember cases in which, after a more or less lengthy period of wavering between alternatives, suddenly something seems to happen interiorly. A decision is made and never changed. It is followed by years of valuable and faithful service in the vineyard of the Lord. On the other hand one will also remember cases of stubborn adherence to attempts to enter the priesthood or the religious life in spite of repeated rejections by Bishops and religious superiors and being told by confessors to remain in the world. The committee of Cardinals formed by Pius X spoke of the importance of a "right intention, along with fitness resting on gifts of nature and grace and proved by uprightness of life and adequate education which will give a well founded hope that the duties of the priesthood will be properly carried out and its obligations holily observed."[10]

---

[8] Taylor's translation, 1924, p. 45.

[9] Words in italics are given only in the *Manuscript* Page 26 right. By the word *Manuscript* in the references her and elsewhere is meant *Les Manuscrits autobiographiques de Sainte Thérèse de l'Enfant Jesus* printed by Draeger Freres (Editions de l'office central de Lisieux, 51 Rue du Carmel Lisieux, France (Calvados). The right and left sides of two opposite pages have only one number, hence the reference above p. 26, right. See Taylor, p. 45.

[10] Guibert, loc. cit., p. 412.

As I remember cases of stubborn persistence I have encountered in the past, the background, thus described by the Cardinals, has been lacking. This stubborn resistance sometimes is indicative of insanity as in the following case: A member of a religious community wanted to join another. He was told that he could not be received. Nevertheless he appeared saying: I have come to stay. He fought viciously against being removed by the police. Nevertheless he kept returning, I think about five times. He gave so much trouble to the local police that finally police from his home state had to come and take him to a mental hospital. Father Robo pictures the fidelity of St. Thérèse to her vocation as something pathological, part of her constitutional psychopathic inferiority, but as we shall see, he misrepresents the facts.

4. The Personal Background to the Vocation of St. Thérèse

Leaving that aside for the present, let any one study the personal. background of the vocation of St. Thérèse as revealed in the first chapters of her autobiography. He will get a very different picture from that outlined by Father Robo.

She lived in a family whose members were outstanding for their sanctity. The members of her family were leading a holy life and she absorbed its principles from them. Spiritual guidance and direction commenced—as it should, but often does not—in the home. St. Thérèse gives us the picture of her childish faults and also of her efforts to correct them. "Mamma, I have pushed Céline. I slapped her once, but I'll not do it again." "It was enough to tell me you must not do that, and I never wanted to do it again."[11]

Very early she learned to practice self-denial. Her mother wrote in a letter in 1876: "Even Thérèse is anxious to make sacrifices. Marie has given her little sisters a string of beads on purpose to count their acts of self-denial. They have really spiritual but very amusing' conversations together."[12] She had already laid the foundation of her *Little Way* and was soon to learn that by self-sacrifice we buy souls for Christ. This would eventually make easy what are really the "little" sacrifices of life in Carmel. Later on she went fishing with her father. "Sometimes I tried my hand with a small rod of my own, but generally I preferred to sit on the grass some distance away. Then my reflections

---

[11]Soeur Thérèse, p. 20. Manuscript, p. 7, right and p. 9, left.
[12]Soeur Thérèse, p. 23.

became really deep, and without knowing what meditation meant, my soul was absorbed in prayer . . . Earth seemed a place of exile and I dreamed of Heaven.[13] As I grew older my love of God grew more and more. I often offered my heart to Him, using words my Mother had taught me."[14]

We must look upon the various stimuli that St. Thérèse experienced in childhood to keep on advancing in spiritual perfection as examples of God's illuminating and inspiring graces. She seems to have made the most of them. Thus while Céline was preparing for her First Holy Communion, she tells us: "One evening I heard someone say to my happy little sister: 'From the time of your First Communion you must begin an entirely new life.' At once I made a resolution not to wait till the time of my First Communion, but to begin with Céline."[15]

We have now presented the background of the spiritual life into which there came the call to enter Carmel that we mentioned above. She tells us how one evening, as we have noted, while thinking over the picture Pauline had given her of religious life: "I felt that the Carmel was the desert where God wished me also to hide. I felt this so strongly that I had not the least doubt about it; nor was it a childish dream, but the certainty of a Divine Call."[16]

Vocations to the religious life sometimes come suddenly. At the same time the one who receives the call feels no longer any doubt about the matter. It takes the form of an obligation that one must carry out, if in any way possible. The degree of certainty as to the divine character of the call varies. In general such calls eliminate any desire to take up any other career and give the person a strong desire to be a priest or to enter a religious community. But in the case of St. Thérèse was this call a manifestation of pathological stubbornness or did it come from God? The Committee of Cardinals mentioned above tells us that for a practical judgment we must examine the personality background in which the call resounds.

We have a candidate that from earliest childhood has been trying to overcome faults, to practice self-denial and do all in her power to attain perfect self-command. God Himself seems to have introduced her to the ways of prayer and seems to have given her at times a taste

---

[13]Loc. cit., p. 32. Manuscript, p. 15, left.
[14]Loc. cit., p. 33-34. Manuscript, p. 16, left.
[15]Loc. cit., p. 44. Manuscript, p. 25, right.
[16]Loc. cit., p. 45. Manuscript, p. 26, right.

of true contemplative prayer. This background seems eminently satisfactory and it may well be that this call at the age of about nine truly came from God. But nine is clearly too young. Is it unreasonable for her when approaching fifteen to seek a dispensation of one year in order to follow her call? One must admit that at fifteen she had a spiritual maturity seldom attained even in the twenties or later.

Let us study what she did in the light of Father Robo's charge of pathological stubbornness.

5. Steps Taken by St. Thérèse to Enter Carmel at Fifteen

We must remember that the main source of guidance and information that St. Thérèse received in the course of the development of her spiritual life was from her family. First of all by example. We may pause to take a glance at that example. "Every morning saw them at Mass; together they knelt at the Holy Table. They strictly observed the fasts and abstinences of the Church, kept Sunday as a day of complete rest in spite of the remonstrances of friends, and found in pious reading their most delightful recreation. They prayed in common, after the touching example of Captain Martin, whose devout recital of the *Our Father* brought tears to the eyes of his hearers. The great Christian virtues flourished in their home. Wealth did not bring luxury in its train, and the simplicity of olden days characterized the household."[17]

Charity to the poor was an outstanding trait. "On one occasion Louis Martin was seen to raise a drunken man from the ground in a busy thoroughfare, take up his bag of tools, support him on his arm, and lead him home. " Another time seeing in a railway station a poor and starving epileptic without the means to return to his distant home, he was so touched with pity that he took off his hat, and, placing in it an alms, proceeded to beg from the passengers on behalf of the sufferer. Money poured in, and it was with a heart brimming over with gratitude that the sick man blessed his benefactor."[18]

In listening to a sermon St. Thérèse tells us: "I must own, I looked at Papa more than at the preacher, for I read many things in his face. Sometimes his eyes were filled with tears which he strove in vain to keep back; and as he listened to the eternal truths he seemed no longer

---

[17]Rev. T. N. Taylor in Prologue to *Soeur Thérèse of Lisieux, the Little Flower of Jesus*, New York, Kenedy, 1924, p. 6.
[18]Op. cit., pp. 6, 7.

of this earth, his soul was absorbed in the thought of another world."[19]

Secondly the main source of her direction in the spiritual life was the instruction she received from her sisters—for her mother died when she was in her fifth year. Marie taught her to make little sacrifices when she was about four. "The feasts!" she writes, "What precious memories their simple words bring to me. I loved them, and my sisters knew so well how to explain the mysteries hidden in each one."[20] After her mother's death Pauline acted as her mother, and Marie took the part of mother for Céline.

Her soul had been prepared by divine grace and her mind turned in her fourteenth year to Carmel. "The Divine Call was becoming so insistent, that had it been necessary for me to go through fire, I would have thrown myself into it to follow my Divine Master."[21] It was only natural that she should first try to gain the approval of the members of her family. She first spoke to Pauline and was given strong support. Marie thought she was too young. But when Céline heard of her hopes she encouraged her to go ahead. She hated to cause pain to her Father and prayed earnestly before she spoke to him on Pentecost Sunday. The tears rolled down his face but he gave his consent and stood by her and helped her till the day she entered.

Father Robo censures her for not having gone to her confessor for direction and quotes the words of her autobiography. "In those days I did not dare to speak of my inner feelings; the road which I trod was so direct, so clear, that I did not feel the need of any guide but Jesus."[22] These words express how she actually felt at the time. This child of fourteen is not laying down a general rule for the guidance of souls. Nor did she have any knowledge of the theological principles of spiritual direction. She would have to have canonical approval at all events and was merely trying to do what she felt called upon by God to do. Canonical superiors who granted her a dispensation would be responsible for the decision.

---

[19]Op. cit., p. 36. Manuscript, p. 18, left.

[20]Op. cit., p. 35. Manuscript, p. 17, right.

[21]Op. cit., p. 78. Manuscript, p. 49, right.

[22]*Soeur Thérèse of Lisieux.* Trans. by Taylor, Kenedy, 1924, p. 77. Quoted by Father Robo in his book *Two Portraits of St. Thérèse,* 2nd Ed., p. 83. See Manuscript p. 49, left. The wording in the manuscript refers specifically to the problem of making known to one's confessor a desire for more frequent communion. The translated text was condensed.

Father Robo is again not telling the whole truth. He is quoting words without taking into consideration their context. In Taylor's translation and more clearly in the fuller account in the Manuscript, it is quite clear that the words quoted by Father Robo do not refer to her vocation but to her practice of going "to Communion as often as my confessor allowed me, but never to ask for leave to go more frequently." She continues these words saying: "Now however I would act differently, for I am convinced that a soul ought to disclose to her director the longing she has to receive her God."[23]

"I needed no other guide but Jesus" was clear, in the matter of more frequent communion, because as a matter of fact the permission needed came from Christ through her director without her having asked. She then passes on to the fact that she felt Our Lord's guidance in her inner life and quotes the canticle of St. John of the Cross "I had no other guide nor light except that which burned within my heart."[24] We all know that St. John of the Cross did not mean by these words that a soul should get along without spiritual direction. Neither did St. Thérèse.

Should a director *always* follow his own ideas about how his patient should act without any consideration of the fact that the Holy Spirit might have given the soul certain lights and impulses?

Consider the following words of Ignatius Menendez-Feigado, O.P. "In questions of obedience the director may easily make mistakes, because sometimes the certitude which God infuses in the soul is so great that no matter how much the soul may desire to obey the director, it cannot help but think that such and such a thing is not so or that it must do a certain thing in the way that has been communicated to it. The director must not confuse this attitude with attachment to one's own opinion; he need but observe carefully to see whether the soul sincerely desires to do what it is told but cannot because the command is contrary to what it has received interiorly."[25]

Father Robo does not allow for the tender years of St. Thérèse in this crisis of her life, nor does he give any evidence of having considered seriously the possibility that God had called her to enter Carmel around about her fifteenth birthday without being obliged to wait till

---

[23]Taylor's translation, p. 77. Manuscript, p. 49, left.
[24]Manuscript, p. 49, right. Full stanza in Taylor, p. 76.
[25]*Cross and Crown*, Qualities of a Spiritual Director, 1950, Vol. 2, p. 183.

she was sixteen or even twenty-one as demanded by the canonical superior of the Carmelites.

Is it clear that in the matter of her vocation she never made known to any priest "the longing she had to enter Carmel"? There is a very beautiful letter reproduced from Thérèse's rough draft in which she did precisely this. True it does not present the matter as it were canonically asking advice and approbation or rejection. It merely tells of her longings and hopes. Father Almire Pichon, S. J., to whom it is directed, was closer to being her spiritual director than any other priest. She tells how her sisters in Carmel had evidently urged her to open her mind to him that he might direct her.[26]

So as the matter stands:

1. The passage referred to by Father Robo as proving rejection of spiritual direction in the matter of her vocation refers to quite another matter: not satisfying her desire for more frequent communion by asking the permission of her confessor.

2. St. Thérèse, at the instigation of her two sisters in Carmel to seek direction from Father Almire Pichon, S. J., wrote to him telling him of her desire and hope of entering Carmel. Had he thought it a grave mistake he should have warned her against it. But there seems to be no record of his answer.

As a matter of fact Père Pichon replied to this letter by a personal visit. Père Pichon, director of both Marie and Céline, was the only one informed of all her plans. "She revealed them to him during a visit he made to Lisieux. He encouraged them unreservedly, including the appeal to Leo XIII.[27]

The superiors of Carmel did not encourage her. She tried to get her uncle's approval and after a preliminary strong opposition he changed his mind and said that after praying to God he felt she was following God's call. "Go in peace, my dear child, you are a privileged little flower which Our Lord wishes to gather."[28] But the canonical superior of the Carmelites said: No; and that she would have to wait until she was twenty-one; and referred them to the Bishop of Bayeux. During

---

[26]Collected letters of St. Thérèse of Lisieux, edited by Abbe Combes. Trans. by F. J. Sheed, New York, Sheed and Ward, 1949, p. 29. On Père Pichon see Stephane-Joseph Piat, Le Pére Pichon *Etudes et Documents* Lisieux, Oct, 1957, *33*, pp. 61-64.
[27]Stephane-Joseph Piat, O.F.M. *The Story of a Family*, New York, Kenedy, 1948, p. 345-346.
[28]Manuscript, p. 52 left. This page is not numbered.

all this time her life went on as usual. "I went on studying, and, what is more important, I went on growing in the love of God. Now and then I experienced what were indeed raptures of love."[29]

The Bishop received them kindly. Her father said they were going to Rome and if necessary would speak to the Holy Father. The Bishop *did not refuse permission,* but said he himself would speak to the Canonical Superior of the Carmelites and they would have his answer while they were in Italy. He said to Thérèse: "All is not lost, little one. Going to Rome will strengthen your vocation."[30] In the audience with the Holy Father, Leo XIII, when it came her turn to kneel before him, she hesitated to speak. Céline said, "Speak." She did so and naturally was merely told: "Do whatever the superiors decide. You will enter if it is God's will."

Thérèse tells us that after her "failure" in Rome: "I felt a deep inward peace, for I had made every effort in my power to respond to the appeal of my Divine Master."[31] That expresses the specific nature of the call that had been given her: Do all you possibly can to enter Carmel at fifteen. She had done it, and was at peace. Had she been driven on by pathological selfishness, the result would not have been peace, but rebellion. Of rebellion there was not the slightest trace.

Furthermore the whole series of efforts was not dictated to her by her own selfishness. She was following the instructions of her spiritual director and also of her "little mother" Pauline.

"In the year that preceded Thérèse's own entry into Carmel, Sister Agnes of Jesus (Pauline) was her chief counsellor and support in her fight to join her in Carmel at the age of fifteen. Writing to her in Rome during the pilgrimage in November 1887, she strongly urged her to put her case before the Holy Father, himself. 'Above all,' she says, 'do not be put off by a first refusal. Think of the perseverance of the Canaanite woman. If the Holy Father seems to say no, say to him, Holy Father, you cannot refuse me, you know that Jesus said, Let the little children come unto me.' "[32]

On December 28, 1888 the Superioress of Carmel at Lisieux received a letter from the Bishop of Bayeux authorizing the immediate entry of

---

[29]Op. cit., p. 82. Manuscript, p. 52, right.
[30]Op. cit., p. 86. Manuscript, p. 55, not numbered, right.
[31]Op. cit., pp. 99-100. Manuscript, p. 64.
[32]Rev. Francis Horsfield," Pauline Enters Carmel," *The Saint of Lisieux,* October, 1952. Vol. 5, No. 2, p. 74.

Thérèse into Carmel. But the Superioress decided to postpone
Thérèse's entry till after Lent, 1889.

Father Robo does not tell the whole truth and nothing but the truth
in his account of her interview with the Bishop. "Nothing can stop her.
She goes to the Bishop, who does not take her seriously, and finally to
the Pope.[33] Her obstinancy and her tears can only be explained by
the conviction that not only was she right, but that she was seeking the
will of God and that her mission was to make every one execute it."[34]

But the Bishop did take her seriously and promised that she would
have his answer while in Italy, as we have just pointed out. But on
December 16th, not having had an answer, she wrote again. Father
Robo, strange to say, did not take the trouble to look at the letter sent
to the Bishop and published in *Collected Letters of Saint Thérèse of
Lisieux*,[35] and quotes from *Bowers, Storm of, Glory;* passages in which
she says that Little Jesus wanted her in Carmel at Christmas and that
it was through the Bishop He was going to fulfil it. He omits to quote
the following words: "Whatever pain a refusal would cause me, I
should accept it with the entire submission, as coming from God
Himself." True, M. Guerin corrected her first rough copy. In the
original she says: "I shall never forget that it is to your Excellency that
I shall owe the accomplishment of God's will" which might be either
approval or refusal. That St. Thérèse had already accepted a refusal
is clear from the peace without rebellion that she experienced after her
apparent failure with the Holy Father. Not to mention her
acquiescence in a refusal from the Bishop is not telling the whole truth.

From this account it would seem that we have every right to look
upon the desire to enter Carmel that St. Thérèse experienced as a call
that came to her from God. In the light of her perseverance until
death and her attainment to sanctity in Carmel and of her canonization by the Church, no other concept is possible. The attempt to
explain her conduct as that of a girl, wilful and disobedient, to a
prodigious degree is a false attribution of selfishness to a holy child.
It is contrary to the evidence in documents available for years. It is an
example of how a historian was not "the servant of the evidence."

If St. Thérèse was, as Father Robo says, wilful and obstinate to a
prodigious degree in the pursuit of her vocation, her calling to Carmel

---

[33]*Two Portraits*, 2nd Ed. p. 84.
[34]Op. cit., 2nd Ed., p. 85.
[35]Collected Letters, p. 41.

was not according to St. Ignatius a vocation which came from God. For as St. Ignatius says: "*Every* divine vocation is always pure and clean without being mixed with fleshly desire or *any other inordinate affection whatsoever.*"[36] The desire of St. Thérèse to enter Carmel at fifteen received the approval of the Bishop of her diocese and her spiritual director. The story of her life tells us that her vocation was something that commenced when she was two years of age. A little later she desired to enter Carmel, not to be with her sisters, but for the sake of Jesus only. She persevered in Carmel until death. She attained therein to the heroic sanctity of the Saints. The Church bore witness to her true sanctity by her canonization and God Himself by the many miracles that have been wrought by her intercession. Her vocation was evidently a call from God.

---

[36]*Exercitia Spiritualia* S. P. Ignatii De Loyola. Latin version by John Roothaan, Augsburg, 1887, p. 175. (Preamble to making an election). Italics in original.

CHAPTER XXII

Did St. Thérèse Suffer A Mental Breakdown?

1. St. Thérèse as a Psychopathic Personality With Psychosis

Let us consider for a moment a question asked by Father Robo: "Why should imfirmities such as neurosis, be greater obstacles than bodily ones? We can even go further. Why should insanity, at least intermittent insanity, make great holiness impossible?"[1] The obvious answer is that there is a difference in insanities.

Take for instance what psychiatrists call reactive depressions, or "the depressive reaction, which is precipitated by a current situation, frequently by some loss sustained by the patient."[2] See for instance the example given above (p. 105ff), of the woman who to gain sympathy, made an attempt at suicide by shooting herself in the abdomen. Would such an attempt at suicide be compatible with heroic sanctity? Would not heroic sanctity demand patient endurance rather than suicide?

Then again the condition termed by many psychiatrists constitutional psychopathic inferiority. One might conjecture that Father Robo has this condition in mind when he speaks of her as a neuropath whose condition resulted in a mental breakdown (a psychosis). But the behavior of St. Thérèse does not warrant the diagnosis. Be that as it may, a constitutional psychopath could not remain what he is and qualify for canonization. "They constitute[3] a rebellious, individualistic group who fail to fit into their social *milieu,* and whose emotional instability is largely determined by a state of psychological immaturity which prevents them from adapting to reality and profiting by experience. They may be adult in years, but emotionally they are

---

[1] *The Two Portraits,* 2nd Ed. p. 229.

[2] Diagnostic and Statistical Manual: Mental Disorders. American Psychiatric Association, 1785 Massachusetts Ave. N.W., Washington, D.C., p. 33.

[3] Sir David Henderson, Gillespie and Bachelor. *A Textbook of Psychiatry.* Oxford University Press. London, 1956, p. 384.

so slow and backward and uncontrolled that they behave like
dangerous children. They lack judgment, foresight and ordinary
prudence."[4]

"The psychopath shows a striking inability to follow any sort of life
plan consistently, whether it be regarded as good or evil. He does not
maintain an effort toward any far goal at all."[5]

Any psychiatrist with considerable experience in the problems of
adolescents and adults will be able to call to mind a number of patients
whom he has attempted to help in whom these two characteristics are
found together as outstanding symptoms of their mental disorder.

Let us now raise the question whether or not a psychopathic
personality could pass the searching scrutiny of the Church and be
proclaimed to have possessed Faith, Hope and Charity to God and
man along with Prudence, Justice, Temperance, Fortitude and their
related virtues in an heroic degree.[6] I think every psychiatrist would
laugh at the very thought of any such thing. A saint's control over
emotions and impulses and power of guiding life to a noble end by the
theological and moral virtues must not merely be outside the region
of pathological defect but at the other extreme, at the very heights of
what is possible to man. To call *a canonized saint a psychopath is therefore
to call in question the judgment of the Church in her decree of canonization.*

There are indeed saints who have gone through psychotic episodes
and have proved their sanctity by the way in which they managed the
extra burden thrown upon them by their mental suffering. But no
psychopathic personality ever was or ever could be canonized by the
Church if you understand by psychopath one who was incapable of
managing his life with the *perfection* of prudence, justice, fortitude and
temperance in accordance with the ideals of Faith, Hope and Charity.

But could one of these constitutional psychopaths cure himself and
then rise to the heights of sanctity. Father Robo seems to have this
very concept in mind when he concludes his book with these words.

---

[4] Psychiatrists of various nations use this phrase. Thus David K. Henderson, *The
Psychopathic Personality*, Oxford University Press, 1952; Kurt Schneider, *Die psycho-
pathischen Persönlichkeiten* (a classic study) in *Aschaffenburgs Handb. der Psychiatrie*,
Leipzig-Wien 1923; Clemente Catalano-Nobili, *La Personalita psychopatische di
Roma Pazz*, 1953; Gustavo Lotteroth-Suarez, *Breve revision del concepto personalidad
psycopatica* Tesis-Univ. d. Mexico, 1952.
[5] Hervey Cleckley, M.D., *The Mask of Sanity*, St. Louis Mosby 1955, p. 417.
[6] Codex of Canon Law, 2104.

"To the praise of St. Teresa, let us point out that a weakness which is usually a life-long handicap was conquered by her as far as one can conquer an incurable infirmity, and that she made an unexpected use of it as the means of reaching sanctity."[7]

But no one can point out a period in the life of St. Thérèse when she was a rebellious, individualistic person who behaved like a dangerous child and was unable to follow any sort of plan or maintain any effort toward any goal at all.

On the contrary, obedience to authority and kindness to all and an unfaltering pursuit of true sanctity were her outstanding traits from earliest childhood to death.

One will get into endless complications if one attempts to take seriously the use of the words neuropath, neurosis and psychoneurosis in *The Two Portraits*. The reason for this probably is that the author is not familiar with their technical meaning. When he says neuropath he must in reality mean psychopath for neuropathy means some kind of injury to the nervous system. But he only speaks of such things as tearfulness, scruples, sadness and other emotional states that have no known dependence on a definitely localized injury or disease of the nervous system.

If one looks upon Father Robo's word *neuropath* as meaning nothing more or less than a person suffering from emotional difficulties and *neurosis* as equivalent to *psychoneurosis* (as it is in fact frequently used) and both to mean a tendency to be more or less emotional then he will have no difficulty in agreeing with Father Robo that a neuropath can be a saint. But he will have difficulty in finding anyone who is not a neuropath and does not suffer from a psychoneurosis.

But the moment one says a neuropath is what psychiatrists formerly termed a constitutional psychopath and finds out the two outstanding symptoms of a constitutional psychopath, he will have great difficulty in agreeing with him that St. Thérèse was a constitutional psychopath, for that diagnosis indicates a person

1. who has no fixed plan in life and is constitutionally unable to follow out any plan to its successful achievement.

2. one who is ever having difficulties in one's interpersonal relations: at home, in school, in business or wherever he may be.

One can, as we shall see, suffer from manic depressive insanity and

---

[7] *The Two Portraits*, p. 238, 2nd. Ed.

various other mental disorders and manifest his sanctity by patient endurance. (See p. 209ff). But one cannot suffer from a constitutional psychopathy in the technical sense and manifest sanctity by giving up one honest position after another, accomplishing nothing and quarrell--ing with all with whom he comes in contact.

Father Robo seems to mean that St. Thérèse suffered from her neuropathy all her life and sanctified herself by dealing with it. She did deal successfully with various emotional conditions. But she

1. was not devoid of any fixed plan in life and she did pursue ends to their successful fulfilment. As to the minor plans, she successfully pursued her studies so as to lead her class when at school. She did overcome her extreme tearfulness. Her one great plan in life was the attainment of sanctity in Carmel. This commenced as early possibly—though in a vague way—in her second year and was pursued unremittingly until her death. Her labors were crowned with success and recognized by the Church on the day of her canonization by Pius XI in 1925.

2. She never had clashes and was never "on the outs" with others at home, or in school or in the convent. Kindliness and friendly sympathy to all was an outstanding trait in all her dealings with others.

St. Thérèse was not a neuropath if by that you mean what was once termed a constitutional psychopath by psychiatrists. But she did have various emotional difficulties. But who goes through life free from emotional difficulties?

The diagnosis of "mental disorder" places a stigma on anyone to whom it is attached. The efforts of psychiatrists have not yet been able to remove the stigma from the diagnosis. It should never be made except by a properly qualified psychiatrist or board of psychiatrists. The custom of the law allowing an ordinary jury to pass on the insanity of a criminal might well be changed and a demand at least be made that an established board of psychiatrists should register an opinion.

It involves at times some intricate problems. We have pointed out above that there is an essential difference between a psychoneurosis with depressive reaction and constitutional recurrent manic-depressive psychoses. Shock therapy is likely to help such psychoses but is usually ineffective in the psychoneurotic condition. (See above p. 130—131). The difficulty of the problem has been thus expressed. "It is important both from the prognostic and the therapeutic point of view to diagnose between, for example a constitutional recurrent depressive, a hysterical type of personality suffering from a largely psychogenic depression, and a comparatively normal type of personality in a state of depression reactive to particular external circumstances."[8]

Father Robo boasts of having been trained in historical research. Does that training enable him to make this difficult differential diagnosis in psychiatry? Furthermore he maintains that in her tenth year she entered into a psychosis. This involves a differential diagnosis between a mental disorder and an acute infection. Does training in historical research give him any competency to make such a differential medical diagnosis?

2. Mental Disorders Compatible With Sanctity

As we have just pointed out, if anyone is a psychopathic personality, he cannot possibly be a saint. But that does not mean that all psychotic conditions are incompatible with sanctity.

Let us study what looks like psychotic episodes in two saints canonized by the Church.

St. Francis de Sales: St. Francis de Sales was sent by his father to make his studies in Paris when he was only 13 years of age. After four years there he had not only studied philosophy and science at the Jesuit College of Cleremont, but had also obtained permission to follow courses in Theology, Sacred Scripture and Hebrew at the Sorbonne.[9]

When about 17 he entered into a state of acute anxiety. It commenced with the thought that perhaps he was not in the state of grace. At the same time he felt weak and lacked spirit and energy. All this weighed upon his mind but he did not break under the burden. He regarded his condition as a temptation and considered it his duty to make issue with it. But then there came as it were a whispering: If you are not in grave sin you would certainly fall into it should a dangerous occasion present itself. He met this by thinking: God never deserts one in the presence of danger.

His tormenting thoughts, however, would not give way to logical conclusions based on revealed truths. Furthermore the sweetness of

[8] W. Mayer-Gross, Eliot Slater, and Martin Roth. *Clinical Psychiatry* Baltimore, Williams and Wilkins, 1956, p. 209.
[9] M. Hamon, *Vie de Saint Francois de Sales*, Paris, Lecoffre, 1875, pp. 43-44.

divine love that he had previously enjoyed was withdrawn. That led
to the thought: perhaps these aridities are due to some hidden sin.
Then there came to his mind the concept, held by some, of the small
number of the elect and the shadowy depths of the concept of predestination. It seemed to him that one as wicked as himself could
never hope to be among the small number of the elect. He replied to
this that even if he were to be damned in the end, he wanted to love
God as long as he could. The thought of hell as a place of blaspheming
God overwhelmed him. And he prayed: "O my Saviour, if I should
go to hell never permit that I should curse Thee and blaspheme Thee."
    In the midst of these mental torments his face became worn and
pale. Jaundice spread over his whole body. He suffered intense pains.
He could scarcely walk. He wobbled when he attempted to stand.
But in spite of all he was faithful to his usual spiritual exercises.
    He turned to the study of theology to find a way out, giving special
attention to St. Augustine and St. Thomas. There he found the
concept of God predestining his saints to glory independently of His
foreknowledge of their good works. This concept only increased his
difficulties. He turned to other good theologians and found the concept
that God's predestination to glory involved the foreknowledge of the
merits and sanctity of His elect. The more he studied the more in-
controvertible this opinion became. He fell on his knees in spirit before
St. Augustine and St. Thomas and asked them to forgive him for
adopting an opinion contrary to their own.
    Not long after this, returning to college in a state of deep depression
he dropped into the Church of Saint Etienne des Grès and prayed
before a statue of Our Lady. Hanging nearby was a tablet on which
was written the *Memorare*. He recited it with great devotion. He asked
God by the intercession of Mary to give back to him his health of body
and mind, made a vow of perpetual chastity, and promised to recite six
decades of the rosary every day. Scarcely had he said these words when
he felt a "movement" in his whole body. Something like a leprous
scab seemed to be detaching itself. He was restored to perfect health.
His mind was set at rest. After six weeks of unheard of suffering he
entered into a profound peace.*

---

*Hamon cites as the basis of this account the life of St. Francis de Sales written by
  his nephew Charles-Auguste de Sales; the life by Jean de Saint-Francois (Jean
  Golu); and the work of P. Talon; and the deposition of Sainte Chantal in the acts of
  the process of canonization of St. Francis de Sales.

This short account of the mental sufferings of a saint shows us the way in which one can manage mental and physical ills and be sanctified in the process. Abnormal states of anxiety and depression are not incompatible with sanctity but when properly managed may lead to an increase in spiritual growth. But the state of a psychopathic personality in which one does not maintain normal and wholesome relations with those with whom he comes in contact is incompatible with sanctity.

St. Francis died from a cerebral hemorrhage. Suppose instead of a large hemorrhage leading to death in a few days, he had suffered from multiple microscopic hemorrhages over a period of many months; and that these resulted in a condition of insanity with marked cognitive defect and change of character. Would that condition in itself alone mean a loss of sanctity and a state of mind incompatible with canonization? Not at all, for that which comes about through no fault of our own does not take away from our past merits, nor mean the loss of sanctity previously attained.

St. Alphonsus: Towards the latter part of his life "St. Alphonsus entered on a state of utter exhaustion. He was completely worn out and deprived of all energy. And there followed such a series of ills that he became a cadaver rather than a living body. He ate little and slept less."[10]

It is worth noting that physical illness preceded and accompanied the state of depression and anxiety that was to follow. Janet speaks of an *abaissement du niveau mental* as the basis of various mental symptoms. Unreasonable possibilities overwhelm the mind that has lost physical vigor, whereas in the full strength of the personality they would receive no attention. It has been found that a physical illness or a surgical operation preceded the first onset of scruples in 39 out of 400 cases studied.[11] This same coincidence of physical illness and the onset of anxiety we noticed in St. Francis de Sales.

The first mental symptom in the disorder that developed from the physical condition of St. Alphonsus was an excessive emotional

---

[10]Antonio Maria Tannoia, *Della vita ed instituto di S. Alfonso Maria de Liguori,* Torino, Marietti, 1857, Book IV, Ch. XXX, p. 699. Tannoia's life of St. Alphonsus is like Boswell's life of Samuel Johnson, based on personal reminiscences.

[11]Joseph J. Mullen, Psychological Factors in the Pastoral Treatment of Scruples. *Stud. Psychol. Psychiat.,* Catholic University of America, Washington, D.C., 1927, I, p. 55.

reaction to the situations of life. There came over him an abnormal sense of being no longer of any use in his community. Seeing the young men go out to their apostolic works no longer filled him with pure joy as in the past. His mind was dominated by a sense of his own personal utter worthlessness. Hearing of the troubles caused the Holy Father by Catholic governments, he exclaimed: "Let us pray to God that He may bring about harmony between the Supreme Pontif and the Catholic powers." "O, the poor Pope," he said almost weeping, "rejected and afflicted by his own very children."[12]

The anguish he suffered on hearing of the calamities of the Church became so acute that those about him tried to prevent his learning anything about such affairs. This state of heightened emotivity to the sufferings of the Church was followed by a period in which he could not rid himself of the thought that he might no longer be in the state of grace and his soul would be lost for all eternity. "Who knows", he exclaimed with tears, "Who knows if I stand in the grace of God and that I shall be saved." "O Jesus mine do not permit me to be damned." "Lord," he repeated weeping, "Do not send me to hell, for in hell you are not loved."[13] That last prayer was as good a proof as one could have that he truly loved God and could not be damned. He was conscious of having in the past consoled many who were in the state into which he himself had fallen; unreasonable scrupulosity. But the things he said to others when he repeated them to himself had no effect.

What interests us most is how a saint reacted to this state of intense and unreasonable anxiety. The condition lasted a year or more.[14] One might say that the essence of his reaction was faith in blind obedience to spiritual direction, complete abandonment of himself to God, and patient endurance of his unreasonable anxiety.

He was no longer able to say Mass nor go without assistance to the chapel. So when he was particularly overwhelmed with the thought of being damned forever he would ask to be taken down to the chapel and there he would spend hours in uninterrupted prayer communing with Our Lord in the Blessed Sacrament. "I want to satiate myself with loving Him," he repeated all on fire with devotion, "I still hope to love Him eternally, even though by my sins I deserve hell."[15]

---

[12]Tannoia, loc. cit., p. 705.
[13]Op. cit., p. 706.
[14]Op. cit., p. 708.
[15]Loc. cit.

Many psychiatrists will read these accounts of St. Francis de Sales and St. Alphonsus, smile and say: Clear cases of manic-depressive psychoses with depression and anxiety. But how often have they seen the full picture presented by St. Francis de Sales and St. Alphonsus in mental hospitals or in patients cared for in private practice?

St. Alphonsus seems to bear the heavy burden of a manic-depressive psychosis with anxiety, and yet he does not break down. There is an inner picture to his life seldom if ever seen in mental hospitals. The outstanding element in this picture is a warm love of God that does not waver and a faith that is not obscured. In spite of all, he says to Our Lord in the Blessed Sacrament: "I still hope to love Him eternally." He has no reason to hope; but hope, as a theological virtue, does not depend on reason but flows from sanctifying grace, a gift of God. And because St. Alphonsus hopes in spite of the way things are presented to his mind, sanctifying grace is alive and not dead and he continues to hope in spite of all.

Furthermore we must remember that there is a devil who goes about as a roaring lion seeking whom he may devour. One who does not realize this can never understand many emotional events in the lives of the saints and of ordinary men. Conditions such as those of St. Francis de Sales and St. Alphonsus are fully compatible with the highest sanctity: but what psychiatrists understand by a constitutional psychopath is not compatible with canonization. What Father Robo terms a neuropath seems to be a person marred by constitutional psychopathic inferiority.

3. The Supposed Mental Breakdown of St. Thérèse

Let us now consider what Father Robo terms the mental breakdown of St. Thérèse to which her neuropathic constitution gave rise. The main points in the description he gave of her illness are as follows:

It was preluded by acute mental suffering caused by Pauline's entering the Carmel on October 2nd, 1882. "At the close of the year 1882 *I began to suffer from constant headaches*, they were bearable, however, and did not prevent me from continuing my studies. This lasted till Easter of 1883."*

Her father went to Paris and confided Thérèse and Céline to the care of their uncle. He spoke one evening of her dead mother with

---

*Here and below important phrases have been italicized that were not italicized in the original. See Taylor's translation. Soeur Thérèse, 1924, pp. 47 ff.

great tenderness. She was deeply moved and cried. "That very evening my headache became acute and I was seized with a strange shivering which lasted all night."

When her father returned from Paris she *was physically so ill that he thought she was going to die.*

On Pauline's clothing day she got up and went out to be present for the occasion. "On reaching home I was made to lie down, though I did not feel at all tired: but the next day *I had a serious relapse, and became so ill that humanly speaking, there was no hope for any recovery.*"

We may take this description as indicating that she was physically very ill.

"I do not know how to describe this extraordinary illness. I said things which I had never thought of. I acted as though I were forced to act in spite of myself; I seemed nearly always to be delirious; and yet I feel certain that I was never for a minute deprived of my reason.[16] Sometimes I remained in a state of extreme exhaustion for hours together, unable to make the least movement, and yet, in spite of this extraordinary torpor, hearing the least whisper. I remember it still. And what fears the devil inspired! I was afraid of everything; my bed seemed to be surrounded by frightful precipices; nails in the wall took the terrifying appearance of long fingers, shrivelled and blackened with fire, making me cry out in terror. One day Papa stood looking at me in silence, the hat in his hand was suddenly transformed into some horrible shape, and I was so frightened that he went away sobbing."

The account I have given here is taken from Taylor's translation as evidenced by the citations. I have also at my disposal the facsimile reproduction of St. Thérèse's manuscript.[17] The translation of Father Taylor must have been based on a text that was rewritten, omitting some details and adding others, no doubt supplied by the memory of her sisters. The evident purpose of this reediting was to make an account easier reading for the general public. One sees no trace of an attempt to make St. Thérèse appear as what is termed a "plaster saint." It is the kind of editing that many authors have experienced at the hands of editors that feel that easy reading will be facilitated by elimination and

---

[16]I remember the case of a man in a delirium after an operation. He pulled at the drains till finally he got them out and did other strange things but at the time he thought that his mind was perfectly clear.

[17]Editions de l'office central de Lisieux, 31 Rue du Carmel Lisieux (Calvados).

reediting. There are many little details in the manuscript that are omitted that seem unimportant to the general reader. The result was a much more interesting book than if the full text of St. Thérèse had been published; and the account is essentially true. The description of the acute onset of her condition after Easter 1883 was curtailed. She and Céline had been left with her uncle and aunt during their father's absence in Paris. Her uncle, during the talk about her mother that caused her to weep so much, said he would try to divert her mind by entertainments. That evening she seemed to her aunt too tired to go out with Céline and her cousins. Her aunt told her to go to bed. "In undressing I was taken with a strange trembling. Thinking that I was cold my aunt covered me up with blankets and hot water bottles. But nothing could stop my shaking which lasted almost all night." This does not look like an acute attack of a mental disorder, but more like the onset of pneumonia,[18] or an acute infection of some kind. "My uncle on returning with my cousins and Céline was much surprised to find me in that condition which he looked upon as very serious ... The next morning he brought in Dr. Notta, who like my uncle diagnosed my illness as very grave and one which he had never seen in a child so young."[19] Had her illness been pneumonia he would have diagnosed it without trouble. But that it was something of a serious physical and not of a mental character is evidenced by the fact that when her father returned from Paris Thérèse was so sick that she could not be taken back to her own home.

The facts as given by Father Taylor in his translation do not warrant the diagnosis of a mental breakdown. The facts as given in the manuscript make any such diagnosis impossible. But will Father Robo give up his fundamental claim that St. Thérèse was a neuropath and "her nervous breakdown was not the starting point of this condition but its manifestation in an acute form?"[20]

The child's delirium passed. May came: "The Little Flower alone drooped, and seemed as though it had withered forever. One day the delirium seemed to return, for she was unable to recognize Marie.

---

[18]At the onset of pneumonia in infants, chills are rare. "Chills are not particularly uncommon, however, at the onset of the infection in older children." Mitchell. Nelson *Textbook of Pediatrics*. Ed. by Waldo E. Nelson, Philadelphia, Saunders, 5th Ed. 1950, p. 972.
[19]Manuscript of "The Springtime History of a Little White Flower", p. 28 left.
[20]*The Two Portraits*, p. 73.

Marie, turning towards the statue of Our Lady, "entreated her with the fervor of a mother who begs the life of a child and will not be refused. Leonie and Céline joined her, and that cry of faith forced the gates of heaven. I, too, finding no help on earth and nearly dead with pain, turned to my heavenly Mother, begging her from the bottom of my heart to have pity on me. Suddenly the statue seemed to come to life and grow beautiful with a divine beauty that I shall never find words to describe. The expression on Our Lady's face was ineffably sweet, tender, and compassionate; but what touched me to the depths of my soul was her gracious smile. Then all my pain vanished, two big tears started to my eyes and fell silently.

They were indeed tears of unmixed heavenly joy."[21]

Father Robo sees in this illness nothing more than a psychotic drama through which runs the one motif: a desire to see her mother who was dead.[22] He sums up his concept as follows:

"The illness of Thérèse was due to a mental disturbance and followed a not unusual pattern. The religious mind of the child created the heavenly picture which alone could bring her comfort and recovery. If we ascribe any objective existence to the transfiguration and the smiling countenance of the statue, we can hardly refuse it to the frightening delusions which had previously visited Thérèse in the course of her illness. As the latter expressed her feelings of danger and lack of protection, so the sight of a heavenly mother, powerful, loving, brought about Thérèse's return to health."[23]

All this pseudo-psychology supposes that Thérèse's illness was purely mental and that she was not suffering from a dangerous physical disorder. The following symptoms point to physical rather than a mental disorder.

1. Continuous headache for about three months demands a differential diagnosis and study of physical as well as mental factors.
2. An acute exacerbation of the headache accompanied by chills (and no doubt followed by fever) points to the acute onset of an infectious disorder.
3. A serious relapse the day after she got up to go to her sister's clothing again points to an infection of some kind.

---
[21]*Soeur Thérèse,* 1924, p. 51.
[22]*The Two Portraits,* pp. 69.
[23]*The Two Portraits,* pp. 69-70.

4. Severe physical prostration with a period of delirium is not found in purely mental conditions and points to a toxic delirium due to an infection.[24]

5. A continuation of this physical prostration accompanied by *intense pain* is again further evidence of a serious physical disorder.

None of these symptoms would be present in a purely mental disorder like hysteria. The picture is not that of a manic attack. Nor was it schizophrenia for in the first period of the chronic stage of infections, she goes about her school work as usual.

What infectious disorder comes into consideration when we consider the five headings just laid down? It is naturally impossible to make a certain diagnosis. But among the possibilities pyelonephritis merits consideration. It *could* account for the whole train of events. But that does not allow us to say that it did. On the other hand a purely mental condition such as imagined by Father Robo cannot account for the whole train of events.

Pyelitis is the medical term for inflammation of the pelvis of the kidney. Practically every pyelitis goes on to and involves also the kidney and is termed a pyelonephritis.[25] Urinary infection comprises 1 to 3 per cent of the problems of pediatric practice. A large variety of organisms are found. These may get to the kidney from the blood, having been taken up by loci of infection in various parts of the body such as adenoids, tonsils, teeth, gums, lungs, gastrointestinal tract and many other sources.[26]

A chronic condition may flare up and give rise to an acute attack. "The history in a large proportion of children examined because of either acute or chronic urinary infection suggests that the acute infection is simply the exacerbation of a process initiated in infancy or early childhood."[27] The three months of severe headache spoken of above might have been due to a slight flare-up of a chronic infection.

"The onset of an acute condition is generally sudden with chilliness followed by fever.[28] There are pronounced gastrointestinal dis-

---

[24]See p. 216 for a description of the symptoms in toxic deliria in all acute infections.
[25]See hereon Meridith Campbell. *Clinical Pediatric Urology.* Phila. Saunders, 1951, Chapter 4, pp. 354-495.
[26]Op. cit., p. 355.
[27]Op. cit., p. 359.
[28]Op. cit., p. 386.

turbances. Intense headache, delirium, convulsions, stupor, coma are frequently observed. Meningitis may arise by transportation of infecting organisms to the coverings of the brain."

At the present day with our methods of chemotherapy and antibiotics, a child of ten suffering from pyelonephritis has a very good chance to recover. But in 1883 the condition often remained undiagnosed. In 1837 P. Rayer discovered its pathology and gave it the name Pyelitis.[29] But by 1896 the true concept was lost and Escherisch looked upon it as a disorder of the bladder.[30] At the present time, it might be said that pyelonephritis would be suspected in any obscure febrile disorder in children; and with modern methods of diagnosis the suspicion would be promptly confirmed or laid aside. In 1883 there was no effective treatment, even if a diagnosis were made, and children seriously ill with pyelonephritis (as Thérèse with that or some other febrile condition) usually died. At all events there was no possibility of a sudden relief of all symptoms and a radical cure by what Father Robo terms: the religious mind of the child merely creating in her own imagination the picture of her heavenly mother. We are not bound to look upon her vision as the natural picture of her imagination, if we regard the strange shapes she saw in her delirium as toxic hallucinations. Only a true miracle could possibly have brought about her sudden cure. Our Lady manifested herself to the child, clothed in her immaculate beauty. The expression on her face was ineffably tender and sweet. She smiled upon an innocent child whom she loved and who had a mission on earth that was to be continued in heaven. And as Our Lady smiled all the child's pain vanished. Two big tears of unmixed heavenly joy started from her eyes and flowed silently down her cheeks. Thérèse was cured.

While faithful to our duty to recognize natural cures as natural, we must not be false to our obligation to recognize and acknowledge the almighty power of God when confronted with a miracle.

Summary

The essentials of Father Robo's procedure may be summarized as follows:

(1) We can get a truer picture of a saint by neglecting supernatural ideals and motives that come from divine grace and keep the analysis of the saint's character on a natural level.

---

[29] *Traite des maladies des reins*, Paris, 1837.
[30] Campbell, op. cit., p. 355.

(2) The technique of this analysis is (i) to interpret the saint's behavior in the light of low selfish motives that occur to the mind of the analyzer; (ii) regard all that the saint may say about her higher spiritual and supernatural motives as subjective errors and false explanations of conduct that is dominantly determined by selfishness. This tendency to attempt to justify unworthy conduct by making up praiseworthy motives that really do not exist, is often termed, in psychiatry, rationalization.

(3) Father Robo makes no critical evaluation of his technique, nor does he express any principle on which it is based. But to give it any validity one must assume as true a false promise, namely: The true determining motivation in human conduct is always selfishness or a similar low type of motive and not anything based on high supernatural or even natural ideals. Father Robo's technique therefore involves something closely akin to the Freudian concept that sexual desire is always present as the determining factor in human conduct.

(4) Father Robo maintains that the vocation of St. Thérèse to enter Carmel was dominated by selfishness, that is by a drive to do her own will in spite of everyone. She was not *vere quaerens Deum,* truly seeking God. She was proud and thought that she alone knew what was the will of God.[31] The whole history of her life is against any such conclusion. But Father Robo rules out all objective evidence as "rationalization," assuming his false premise that the true determining motive of human conduct is always selfishness or a similar low type of motive. Father Robo says of such motives: "They are the driving power behind all human activities, and lacking it we should lead the inert life of the sloth in his tree."[32] Freud maintains the same thing of sexuality.

(5) Father Robo diagnoses St. Thérèse as a *neuropath.* But seeing that he mentions no disorders of the nervous system but only mental symptoms his concept must be expressed in the terminology of present day psychology by the word *psychopath.*

But St. Thérèse, throughout her life, manifested nothing like those violent personality clashes that characterize the constitutional psychopath. Furthermore from early childhood until death she consistently pursued one single aim: Sanctity in Carmel. Inability to pursue any aim consistently is the outstanding symptom of psychopaths.

---

[31] *The Two Portraits,* p. 83.
[32] *The Two Portraits,* p. 79.

(6) Father Robo's claim that St. Thérèse suffered a mental break-down collapses completely when we consider facts in her published autobiography. The Manuscript of her life makes it perfectly clear that what Father Robo terms a mental breakdown was a physical illness, due to an infection of some kind starting with chills, accompanied by severe pain and extreme physical prostration and leading, as many infections do, to a toxic delirium.

(7) It is pointed out in the text that Father Robo's position that innate inclinations, unreasoned instincts lurking in the recesses of the unconscious "are the driving power behind all human activities and lacking it we should lead the inert life of the sloth on his tree"[33] is incompatible with (a) the distinction made by St. Thomas Aquinas and Catholic philosophy between sensory and intellectual desires and (b) the teaching of the Church on the illumination of the intellect of man and the inspiration of his will by the Divine Grace.[34]

---

[33] *The Two Portraits*, p. 79.
[34] One will find a sympathetic study of the lifework of Father Robo by C. Marc'hadoux in *Revue des Facultes Catholiques de l'ouest*, 1958, No. 2.

My critique of his *Two Portraits* was undertaken because it seemed to read into the life and character of St. Thérèse of Lisieux much that was derived from her critic's emotions and was, furthermore, only a partial presentation of critically important, available facts. And then the critique could only be made by one who had a background of training in medicine, psychiatry and the spiritual life.

The data of the life of St. Thérèse of Lisieux do not warrant the diagnosis that she ever suffered from a psychosis, or that she had a psychoneurosis or, least of all, that she was a case of constitutional psychopathic inferiority.

Her life cannot be divided into two periods: in the first of which, suffering from a mental disorder, she was "wilful and obstinate to a prodigious degree"; and the second in which she commenced to become a saint by struggling to overcome her mental disorder. She suffered no mental disorder, but bore up heroically under the severe trial of her mother's death when she was somewhat over four years of age.

Heroic Sanctity and Insanity was written not only as an introduction to the spiritual life and as a text on mental hygiene, but also to present a true picture of St. Thérèse of Lisieux. The author regrets that in so doing it was necessary to call attention to a false philosophy and psychology of the human mind, incompatible with fundamental principles in Catholic Theology.

Epilogue

SANCTITY AND MENTAL DISORDER

OUR STUDY OF the Heroic Sanctity of the Saints shows clearly that in mental disorders that may be traced in some way to mental factors, genuine sanctity has prophylactic value. It draws the "would-be" schizophrenic out of himself in to a life of action for God and the welfare of man. It tempers the sadness and unreasonable gaiety of the manic-depressive temperament. It makes more or less impossible the foolish self-pity and even suicidal display of the reactive depression. (See case history p. 105ff).

If sanctity is attained in early life it renders juvenile delinquency impossible. If it reigns in a home it produces peace and contentment. Where charity dominates all, divorce never enters in.

The citizen who is truly holy serves God and gives to Caesar all that is his due. In time of war the man that is holy rises to his duty and risks his life in defense of his country. (See the account of Joyce Kilmer, p. 146ff).

Sanctity does not directly prevent brain disorders due to specific infections and intoxications. But even a moderate degree of holiness may suffice to ward off mental disease due to syphilis. Thus Kraepelin wrote: "Krafft-Ebing saw not a single Catholic priest in 2,000 cases of paresis, but on the other hand, found that as many as 90% of [insane] officers in the army were paretics. Up to the present, paretic nuns seem never to have been observed."[1]

The ultimate reason for the mental hygiene value of sanctity is that it develops a strong and stable personality. A strong and stable personality is one whose mind harbors the ideals of the virtues and who is capable of carrying out these ideals in the stress and strain of daily life. This is something quite different from a stubborn personality. Stubbornness is a drive to carry out personal desires regardless of consequences or whether or not desire harmonizes with virtue.

---

[1] *Psychiatrie*, Leipzig, 1915, 8th Ed., II, p. 437.

221

If sanctity has the mental hygiene value we have just outlined, and it has, psychiatrists should be interested in its development. But one says sanctity can only be utilized in *treatment* when it exists; and it seldom exists in patients that come for psychiatric treatment.

If one will consider the following case history, he will see that the patient was anything but holy. Nevertheless on his own initiative he commenced to lead a good moral and spiritual life and cured himself of a complex of serious mental conditions.

Some years ago a patient came to me, not for treatment, but to tell me how he had cured himself. He was both homosexual and alcoholic. He was also sadistic and masochistic in imagination. Then he had a fetish: he was sexually excited by seeing men's underwear. After reading my book *Personal Mental Hygiene* he got the idea that "religion is the solution for every mental disease."[2] He resolved to commence to lead a devout life. He went to confession and started to go to Holy Mass and receive Communion every day. The result was surprising. Having been homosexual since about nine years of age and having had various affairs with boys and having indulged excessively in alcohol for over twenty years, he soon freed himself entirely from both homosexuality and alcohol. He said that he was now leading a fairly happy life. He had started to take a girl out about once a week. While she would take some kind of alcoholic beverage, he contented himself with a soft drink.[3]

This interesting case suggests that religious therapy need not be confined to those who are already holy. If a man, in whom sanctity is conspicuous by its absence, can on his own initiative commence a devout and holy life and overcome long standing homosexuality and alcoholism, would it not be worth while, at least in some cases, to lead the patient on to a stage in which one might suggest that he commence to lead a truly devout life? Is not this merely one step beyond the starting point in the treatment by Alcoholics Anonymous: "You must get down on your knees and ask God to help you."

After a careful study of the patient, perhaps with dream analysis or other methods of analysing the unconscious, at some subsequent interview the psychiatrist might turn to his patient and say: Look

---

[2] The author does not take this extreme position.
[3] T. V. Moore, *The Nature and Treatment of Mental Disorders*, New York, Grune and Stratton, 2nd Ed. 1951, p. 339 ff.

here: do you want to come out of the mess you are in? Then you must commence by getting down on your knees and asking God to help you.

If this suggestion is not rejected one might go on and suggest a devout life. A Catholic patient might eventually be told to make out for himself a rule of life in which the following elements should find a place: Holy Mass and Communion daily; Confession once a week; Mental Prayer; a visit to a Church and prayer before the Blessed Sacrament— perhaps on returning from work; reading of books on the spiritual life.[4] A simple method of mental prayer is this: Commence reading the four gospels, read and think what can this mean to me in my daily life; turn to God and ask the grace to understand and *do*; from time to time silently love and adore Him Who is always and ever will be everywhere. One should try to find fifteen minutes or a half an hour daily for such prayer. But one exercises mental prayer during Holy Mass and many have no time for more.

Our patient is an example of the truth of what Saint Alphonsus Liguori says about mental prayer: "All the saints were made holy by mental prayer; and we know by experience that those who devote themselves to mental prayer are not likely to fall into mortal sins. But if perchance they do fall, by persevering in prayer they recover their senses and return to God. Mental prayer and sin cannot exist together. . . . One either gives up prayer or stops sinning. But if one does not omit his prayer, he not only quits sinning but turns from the love of creatures to the love of God."[5]

There have been psychiatrists who have looked upon all forms of religion as a psychoneurosis; and therefore felt it their first duty to eliminate the patient's religion if he had any. But that day is passing and there is a well developed movement to bring about active co-operation between psychiatrists and members of the clergy. A psychiatrist leading a devout life himself might well give a patient the suggestions we have just outlined. But one who is not leading such a life might well refer the patient for cooperative help to a sympathetic priest.

---

[4] For example of how a day laborer follows the program. See T. V. Moore, *The Life of Man with God*. Harcourt Brace, New York, 1956, p. 4 ff.

[5] *Praxis Confessarii* Ch. X, III 227, p. 628 in Vol. IV of his *Theologia Moralis*, Rome, 1912.

COOPERATION BETWEEN RELIGION AND PSYCHIATRY

A. The Psychiatric Program
The program of psychiatry at the present day has been thus outlined:
"With the decline of religion and humanism at the turn of the century,
the psychiatrist has moved into a unique position. He is now the
recognized, scientifically trained expert on personality development
and is expected to fulfil all functions previously divided among
clergymen, educators, parents and other agencies . . . At the present
moment of history, many patients cannot accept what religion has to
offer. These individuals consider the psychiatrist to be the only firm
reliance in the ocean of emotional currents. Therefore the present role
of the psychiatrist seems to be to make it possible for the patient to
interact with his social and cultural environment."[6]
The technique of carrying out this program is suggested in the
following words: "Man lives primarily in the cage of his emotional
experiences, and is unable to break the bars of this cage except through
the guidance of other individuals who provide a new viewpoint and
help change unconscious reaction patterns."[7]
It would seem that these passages represent the concept of the
function of psychiatry in the minds of many members of the profession.
But what proportion of psychiatrists hold this concept is unknown.
It is evidently impossible for psychiatrists to carry out the program.
How can a few thousand psychiatrists carry on their own functions and
those of clergymen, educators, parents and other agencies in the
development of personality in all the citizens of the United States.
This becomes clearly evident when one considers the expense per hour
of treatment in a long series of interviews.
It is worth while noting also that while man is the only intellectual
being on the face of the earth, the only one capable of moral ideals and
virtuous conduct, all men are conceived of as being in a cage of
emotional experiences unable to use their own intellect and will like
the patient we have just cited.

---

[6] Dr. Clemens E. Benda. Discussion in Symposium No. 5 *Some Considerations of Early
Attempts in Cooperation between Religion and Psychiatry.* Group for the Advancement
of Psychiatry Publications. Office 1790 Broadway, New York 19, N. Y., March
1958, p. 340.
[7] Loc. cit., pp. 339-340. The quotations do not necessarily represent the personal
opinion of Benda.

How can others cooperate with psychiatrists in their vast and impossible task?

(1) Some clergymen have tried to learn a little about psychiatry and psychoanalysis and act as psychiatrists in dealing with the problems of their parishioners. This type of cooperation has been frowned down upon by American psychiatrists, though *properly qualified* lay-analysts have been in general welcomed in Europe.

(2) The more reasonable program of teaching theological students to recognize mental disorder and refer mental patients to a psychiatrist.

(3) But the following program is more in accordance with priestly work. "I glimpse a rich source, for psychiatry, of able, willing people who are in an excellent position to do not only the job of religious work which psychiatry cannot do, but also deal with certain psychiatric problems so well that they need never reach the psychiatrist."[8]

From what has been said already in *Heroic Sanctity and Insanity* it is clear that this passage may be interpreted as meaning that if all clergymen lead a devout spiritual life themselves and do their duty in leading others to God by the pursuit of all the virtues in a devout spiritual life, the sanctity of many souls will rise to its therapeutic value and be a successful prophylactic agent in preventing mental disorders that might otherwise have risen.

In this sense the Church has but to follow out its usual work for the sanctification of souls to prevent many from developing a mental disorder.

B. The Religious Program

Is there any danger that priests and curates in the confessional or in the parlor will undertake the specific work of psychiatrists and treat mental disorders by various forms of psychotherapy? Any one who knows the busy life of priests working in a parish will see that this will be ruled out by mere lack of time.

Will some priests qualify in medicine and psychiatry and do strictly psychiatric work? Some priests have done so and it may be that others will continue to do so. But that does not mean that the Church will give up its former pastoral work and enter the field of psychiatry, any more than the fact that if some priests teach mathematics or write poetry the Church is deserting pastoral work.

---
[8] Dr. Royden C. Astley, loc. cit., p. 333.

If you would go through the case histories in the files of any psychiatrist you would find some that did not involve moral problems, or
perhaps matters of faith. On the other hand you would find many
that did. Moral problems are common, either as incidental, or as
entering into the very core of a psychoneurosis and behavior difficulties
in adolescence. Psychiatrists are stepping forward as the moral guides
of humanity. Can the Church quietly hand over to the psychiatrists
its duty to define what is sin and what is not sin and to do all in its
power, with the help of God, to keep all men from sin and lead them
to a virtuous life? That will never happen.

Some psychiatrists today say with Freud "we have found it impossible to give our support to conventional sex morality";[9] and do
urge as a relief from the tensions of the moral conflict free indulgence
practised with care. And while some psychiatrists feel that they are
"scientific experts on personality development," I know of none who
outlines the goal of the perfect man who has attained to the height of
virtue in all fields.

This condition of things will probably lead to the development by
the Church of properly staffed psychiatric guidance centers for
children and adults.

But any such development of guidance centers will be but a part of
the sublime program of the Church to lead all men to the perfection of
Faith, Hope, Charity and the moral virtues. What that means in
detail has been outlined in the first part of this book.

The Church has been carrying out that program since the day when
Christ said to His infant Church: "All power is given to me in heaven
and on earth. Going, therefore, teach ye all nations: baptizing them in
the name of the Father and of the Son and of the Holy Ghost,
teaching them to observe all things whatsoever I have commanded you.
And behold I am with you all ways even to the consummation of the
world." (Matthew XXVIII:18-20).

Nearly two thousand years have elapsed since that command and
the pageant of the saints down throughout the centuries bears some
witness to its fulfilment. But the saints are only picked examples.
They had many followers: some even more holy than themselves.

How does the Church carry out its mission to lead all men to the
perfection of virtue?

---

[9] Sigmund Freud, "Introductory Lectures on Psycho-Analysis". London. Allen and
Unwin, 1922, Part III, Lecture xxiii, Transference p. 362.

First of all we may mention the preaching on Sundays. Then the
special missions given from time to time in parishes. Then the retreats
where members of the laity go to some religious house for a week,
follow spiritual exercises, attend conferences and have an opportunity
to speak with the priest who gives the retreat.

But the most extensive source of personal spiritual instruction is the
confessional and the main source of spiritual strength is Holy Mass and
Communion. Many go to Mass and receive Holy Communion daily.
The other sacraments of the Church are channels of grace from on
high.

Then we should mention the oblates of St. Benedict and the various
third orders. Their members live according to a simple rule and have
meetings regularly. The Benedictine oblates go back to the early
middle ages. Members of the laity living around a monastery became
oblates and lived a life of piety. St. Francis of Assisi founded his
Tertiaries in Italy in 1221. The "Third Order" of St. Francis took the
spiritual life to the poor in all regions and was ever very numerous. At
the present time there are some 130,000 Franciscan Tertiaries in the
United States and about three and a half million in the world. There
are eight "Third Orders" in the United States with a membership of
about 200,000.

And then most important of all are the many, many homes throughout our land that are truly schools of the service of God. Here and
there among them are to be found some thousands[10] of adults who have
never been false to God and virtue by a single grievous sin.

Then there are in the United States over 50,000 priests; over
160,000 Sisters; and some 9,000 brothers: an army of some 220,000
who in one way or another consecrate all their energies to helping
others and by prayer and work try to lead all to the development of
their personalities by the practice of virtue.[11]

Those who think that psychiatrists are now called to fulfill all

---

[10]This estimate is based on the results of a questionnaire published in T. V. Moore,
The Life of Man with God, New York, Harcourt Brace, 1956, pp. 386-391.
[11]One should mention here the *Secular Institutes*: societies of priests or members of
the laity who strive to attain to spiritual perfection and carry on an apostolic activity
while living in the world a life of poverty, chastity and obedience. They were
first authorized by Pius xii by an Apostolic Constitution in 1947. For a description
of those existing in North America see J. E. Haley, C.S.C., Apostolic Sanctity in
the World, Notre Dame University Press, 1957, pp. 151—195.

functions previously divided among clergymen, educators, parents and other agencies should pause and count up the costs. Psychiatry is not equipped for any such program.

Should a psychiatrist of this school read this little book on *Heroic Sanctity and Insanity*, he might well compare in his mind the two programs.

(1) One based on the concept: "Man lives primarily in the cage of his emotional experiences, and is unable to break the bars of the cage except through the guidance of others." This centers therapy on emotional life to the exclusion of intelligent responsible action and the development of sanctity.

(2) Man is an intelligent and responsible being. In the ordinary course of events he is educated at home in the school and college and perhaps in the University. He belongs to the universal society in which God is the transcendently Supreme Intelligence in a world of intelligent beings. Because he is necessarily a member in this society his mind is illumined by the true light which enlighteneth every man who cometh into the world. He who is obedient to this light attains to the height of virtue and is spared many ills both mental and physical. Nevertheless he may need from time to time help from a physician and also from a psychiatrist.

Even Aristotle recognized that virtue which comes from philosophy makes a man independent to a large extent of the vicissitudes of life. But he says the philosopher cannot endure the sorrows of Priam. But he who rises from the virtues to the beatitudes can live on in charity with God and man in trials where neither philosophy nor psychiatry can be of any help.

Appendix

1. Current Theories of the Nature of Mental Disorders

We may enumerate under the following headings the various possibilities that have been thought of as the basis of the major psychoses: the manic depressive and the schizophrenic groups of mental disorders.

1. "A mental disorder is an abnormality of human behavior whose specific manifestations depend on the *mental history* of the patient. The character of these manifestations is, therefore, *independent of the original physical constitution or mental temperament of the patient.*"[1]

This concept seems to be implied in the technique and objective of psychoanalysis. A psychoanalyst of our day writes: "A psychoanalyst who might be asked to give very briefly the essential principles of psychoanalysis could say that the recognition of the significance of childhood history for personality development, the teachings of transference and resistance and above all the establishment of the unconscious as an integral part of the human mind constitute the essence of psychoanalysis."[2]

By *transfer* is meant that in the process of psychoanalysis the patient directs to the analyst the feelings he had in childhood, such as love or hate for father or mother. *Positive* transfer is transfer of love. *Negative* transfer is transfer of hate. By *resistance* is meant the opposition that the patient has to allowing the analyst to peer into his unconscious. Perhaps a more general expression of the same phenomena would be the concept of the parataxes: the drive of the mind to perpetuate the emotion which dominates: if sad to stay sad; if angry to stay angry; if it hates to keep on hating.

The accentuation of the importance of the emotional history of

---

[1] The Nature and Treatment of Mental Disorders, New York: Grune and Stratton, 1951, p. 26.

[2] Frieda Fromm - Reichmann, Psychoanalytic and General Dynamic Conceptions of Theory and Therapy. *J. Amer. Psychoanal. Ass.*, 1954, 2, p. 711.

childhood leads psychoanalysts to neglect the significance of the conflict of the present. And concentration on the sexual leads to failure to recognize that other emotions may be at the root of the patient's difficulties. Perhaps the psychiatrists who recognize the necessity of considering the factors neglected by Freud and who are sometimes termed "dynamic" therapists are more numerous today than pure Freudians.

2. Carl Gustav Jung (Born 1875) accentuates the *history of the race*, making the events of childhood and of later life of minor importance. In man there is according to Jung not only a *personal*, but also a *collective* unconscious. The collective unconscious is the inheritance of the experience of primitive man and of the whole human race. It was never conscious in any living man.

From the collective unconscious, man inherits certain drives to react to the problems of life in a special manner. These drives Jung calls *archetypes*. The brain of man today reproduces the archetypes of antiquity.[3]

The concept is so difficult to conciliate with the biological facts of heredity that it has found little resonance in the psychotherapy of our era.

3. A mental disorder is an abnormality of human behavior whose specific manifestations depend largely on the *original physical constitution* of the individual. The work of Ernst Kretschmer on the relation of body build to the types of psychosis might be looked upon as exemplifying this concept. But he recognizes also a relation between the traits of the prepsychotic character and the *mental* symptoms of the psychosis.

4. A mental disorder is an abnormality of human behavior whose specific manifestations depend largely on the original *mental temperament* of the individual. Such a concept is part of the truth. For it has been demonstrated that the symptoms of the major mental disorders are associated with traits in the character of the patient prior to the onset of the mental disorder.[4]

5. A mental disorder is an abnormality of human behavior whose

---

[3] See C. G. Jung, *Psychological Types*, London, 1923. Also a brief digest in T. V. Moore, *The Nature and Treatment of Mental Disorders*, pp. 55-64.

[4] T. V. Moore, The Prepsychotic Personality and the Concept of Mental Disorder. *Character and Personality*, 1941, 9, 169-187.

specific manifestations depend neither on the physical constitution nor the mental temperament of the patient, but on the accidental *localizations of vascular, toxic or other types of cerebral lesions.*[5] The fact that a relation between the symptoms of the major mental disorders and the traits of the prepsychotic character has been established, eliminates this theory of the origin of the major mental disorders. For if such lesions "adequately accounted for the phenomena of the psychoses, the form taken by the psychoses should bear no more relation to the prepsychotic character than disabilities due to gun shot wounds bear to the temperaments existing in the wounded prior to being shot."[6] For if one thing is found with definite frequency whenever another thing is found, they are related by law, but if there is no tendency for them to be found together, their simultaneous occurrence is due to chance. The principle that all mental disease is brain disease was dominant in psychiatry before the days of Freud. Freud's chief merit lies in his successful opposition to this false principle. But unfortunately he went too far in the opposite direction. There are a large number of acute and chronic brain disorders; but there are also a number of psychotic disorders in which mental factors play an important part and in which no pathological condition of the brain has been established by the microscope.

6. A mental disorder is an abnormality of human behavior dependent to a very large extent on the *original psychosomatic constitution* of the patient. This original psychosomatic constitution is manifested by (1) *anthropological* and (2) *mental* traits which tend toward one type of grouping in some individuals and toward quite a different type in others. This concept is the same as that of Kretschmer, except that it accentuates the psychosomatic unity of body and soul.

A study of these six principles will orient us in understanding the origin of the major mental disorders: the essential psychoses. The sixth principle seems to be in accord with empirical investigations. It suggests that a major psychosis is the result of the stress and strain of life impinging on a character that was originally impaired by heredity or which was not duly strengthened and developed by training and sound mental hygiene.

---

[5] Thus for instance P. Blonsky, *Z.f.d. ges. Neurol. u. Psychiat.*, Berlin, 1930, 129, 51-64. Blonsky builds on an earlier concept of Kraepelin, *Z. Neurol.*, 1920, 62.

[6] T. V. Moore, *The Nature and Treatment of Mental Disorders*, New York: Grune and Stratton, 1951, p. 27.

2. Emotional Shock and the Origin of Mental Disorders

Can a sudden emotional shock bring on a psychotic condition? Krafft-Ebing writing from a wide breadth of experience says: "Emotions can without doubt give the impulse which gives rise to a psychotic condition, just as they are occasionally the cause of hysteria, epilepsy, chorea, paralyses, aphasias, and can even result in death through a kind of shock paralysis of the heart and respiration. Again, on the other hand, they can bring about a cure of a mental condition: a paralysis of volitional activity, aphasic conditions, etc."[7]

An actual case will give us a better picture of what happens in a mental disorder due to profound emotional shock:

"The patient was a girl almost 13 years of age when she was brought to the clinic for auditory and visual hallucinations, and a delusion that her touch was poisonous and had killed her mother's cousin, who in reality died of cancer.

"Prior to the manifestation of these symptoms she was said to have been a perfectly normal child.

"Some two or three months prior to the appearance of the girl's symptoms,[8] her little 7-year old brother was digging a tunnel in a sand pile and a big boy ran up and jumped on the mound, and caved in the tunnel. When the little boy was dug out he was dead. This was a profound shock to the patient and she kept brooding over her little brother's death, during a period in which the family noticed nothing abnormal about her conduct.

"Some weeks after her little brother's death, while reading in the newspaper the story of two murderers, she became obsessed with the idea that she might kill someone. Then she heard that her mother's cousin had died of cancer, the thought came to her mind that she had touched the flowers that her mother had brought to her cousin when she was ill. Then came the idea that her touch had contaminated the flowers with poison, and that poison from her fingers had been the real cause of her cousin's death.

"When she came to the clinic she had the idea that she had poison all over her dress, so that if anyone touched her, he might die of the poison. She tormented her father by insisting that he wash and rewash his hands.

[7] R. von Krafft-Ebing, *Lehrbuch der Psychiatrie*, Ed. 7, Stuttgart, 1903, p. 162.
[8] In Krafft-Ebing's experience there is a latent period between the emotional shock and the appearance of the mental disorder.

"Along with these abnormal anxieties there developed crying spells lasting for an hour or so at a time and coming on about once a week. But several spells would usually occur on the day on which one appeared. The patient complained of pain in the epigastrium at these times and tormented her mother with questions.

"Besides her delusional concepts, the child seems to have experienced something akin to visual and auditory hallucinations. She would at times see, or rather as she expressed it "not exactly see," electric chairs and chains, as if someone were going to try 'to get me and tie me up with chains.' Then again she would seem to hear a voice that said 'Francis (her little brother who was killed in the sand pile) is in heaven.'

"At times she was negativistic to her mother's requests. Her expression was dreamy and somewhat expressionless. She was said to have muttered and mumbled to herself at times and was once found talking to herself. Several times a day she was a source of anxiety to her mother because of what were termed 'spells of crossness' lasting half an hour or more. There was no euphoria and no retardation. Her general mood was one of anxiety conditioned by delusions. Sadness, strictly speaking, was not markedly in evidence at any of her visits to the clinic. Besides her anxiety about poison, the patient had a chronic fear of dogs."[9]

Dream analysis revealed that the child thought that her mother had been unkind to her. "Maybe" she said, "I killed my real mother when I was born." Functioning in her mind were ideas from fairy tales: the killing of a little girl with an apple flushed with poison and tales of stepmothers. The patient was given to day dreaming about such things as the pretty clothes she might wear if she had fifty dollars.

Psychotherapy of both child and mother led to a rapid clearing of symptoms. Within a month she was no longer troubled with the delusional fear of poisoning others by her touch.

She was seen fifteen years later. She had a good position, was a healthy happy woman, still single, and during the interim she had had no return of the mental trouble of her childhood.

We will not discuss the problem further than to say that emotional shock may have a physical as well as a mental resonance and therefore in major psychoses both physical and mental factors may be involved

---

[9] T. V. Moore, *The Nature and Treatment of Mental Disorders*, New York: Grune and Stratton, 1951, pp. 79-81.

in varying proportions; for man is not two substances, a body and a soul, but one psychosomatic organic substance vivified by a soul.

The question arises: Could the illness suffered by St. Thérèse in 1882 when she was nine years old have been a psychogenic mental disorder. Several things rule this out: (a) The onset with chills throughout the night no doubt accompanied by fever as such chills are. (See p. 213ff.). (b) Profound physical prostration such as one suffers in an acute infectious disorder. (c) The mental symptoms with clouding of consciousness and inability to recognize her sister and her father and hallucinations of a characteristic terrifying nature and various other things such as a relapse on getting up and going out, make it quite evident that she was suffering from an infectious disorder with delirium. The picture is quite different from the emotional psychotic reaction we have just described: no chills and fever, no physical prostration, no clouding of consciousness with inability to recognize persons about her.

3. Can Chronic Emotional Strain Bring On a Psychotic Condition?

A very suggestive series of observations is the fact that the *percentage* of first admissions to New York State hospitals in whom financial loss was considered as a possible factor rose rapidly from 2 in 1929, the year of the great financial crisis, to over 9 in 1934 and then sharply declined. Very much the same type of rise is found in manic-depressive and dementia praecox first admissions, only that the rise commences with an abrupt ascent in the very year of the depression, 1929.[10]

Evidence of the effect of chronic stress and strain on the onset of psychotic conditions is also to be found from the stastistics published in the annual report of the commissioner of mental disease in Massachusetts.

The rate of total first admissions and readmissions in Massachusetts in 1934 for 100,000 of the population was for the single 261·1; for the married 158·83; for the widowed 330·93; for the divorced 745·1.

The higher rate for the single might have various explanations; but it would seem that the stress and strain of life more than doubles the insanity rate for the widowed over that of the married. The very high rate for the divorced probably means that they were divorced because

---

[10]See the curves given in T. V. Moore, *The Nature and Treatment of Mental Disorders*, 1951, pp. 85-86. Based on the work of Benjamin Malzberg. "The Influence of Economic Factors on Mental Health". *Am. A. Advancement of Sc. Publ.* No. 9, 1939, 185 ff.

they were insane rather than that they became insane because they were divorced.

4. Can a Type of Life Reduce the Insanity Rate?

The Massachusetts data on the insanity rate in the single, married, widowed and divorced compared with that of priests, sisters, and lay brothers is as follows:[11]

Rates per 100,000 in Massachusetts		Total Number of		Rates per 100,000
Single	261·6	Priests, secular and		
Married	158·83	religious	30,250	121·65
Widowed	330·73	Sisters, active and		
Divorced	745·1	cloistered	122,220	124·40
		Brothers, lay and in		
		communities	7,408	69·65

If one examines the above table he will see that the insanity rates per 100,000 of Priests and Sisters in the United States in 1935 were distinctly lower than for the married in the general population. The first question that arises is whether or not the difference is *significant*. I calculated the standard error of the difference in two ways, one by getting from the United States census for Massachusetts the number of married men and women in Massachusetts in 1930 and 1940. I took the mean as the number for 1935. Then from the Annual Report of the Commissioner of Mental Diseases for the year ending 30 November 1934 (The Commonwealth of Massachusetts) I calculated the total number of married men and women from the insanity rates as given in the report. Then having the total number of Priests and Sisters, I

[11]See: Insanity in Priests and Religious, *Am. Eccles. Rev.* 1936, *95*, p. 490 and p. 486.
It would be well to note here that the rate per hundred thousand is based on the sum of the First Court Admission, Court Admissions and All Temporary Admissions. The reason for this is that my data for priests and religious were for all admitted in the year 1935 regardless of any distinctions. In comparing the rates for priests and religious for rates of single, married etc. in various studies, one will find that the rates in some studies are distinctly lower. The reason for this is that at times rates have been given based only on first court admission or on all court admissions exclusive of other temporary admissions, etc.

calculated the standard error of the difference of a proportion: the proportion of insane to all normals.*

In the first case the ratio of the difference to the standard error of the difference was over 3·00 and in the other over 4·00. Seeing that anything over 3·00 is regarded as certainly significant, there must be some reason other than chance to account for the fact that the insanity rate in priests and religious is lower than that of the married, who have the lowest rate in any marital class of the general population.

What could account for the difference? The first thing to ask is: Were my rates low because I did not get full data from all mental hospitals? Information was obtained from 100% of the Catholic hospitals, 96.53% of the state institutions, 100% of the city hospitals, 91.04% of the county sanatoria, and 76.96% of the private institutions."[12] A correction was applied raising the numbers found on the basis of the ratio of the percentage found, answering to the percentage of the whole. It was negligible. Seeing that the state hospitals do not contain all the married men and women in Massachusetts with mental disorders our data were more complete than that of the Annual Report.

Is the lower insanity rate in priests and sisters due to security as to food, clothing and shelter? A man serving a life sentence in prison has the security but he lives an unhappy life under stress and strain.

A study of the present work will show that a devout life has a tendency to prevent many psychogenic mental disorders. A study of the author's work *The Life of Man with God* will show that many priests and nuns do attain to a beautiful spiritual life which may be taken as illustrating sanctity at its therapeutic level. It would seem that there are enough priests and nuns who rise to the therapeutic level of sanctity to lower their insanity rate.

But what is true of priests and religious is also true of holy souls in the world. Their sanctity rises to true heroism and they say with St. Paul: God forbid that I should glory, save in the Cross of our Lord, Jesus Christ." (Gal. VI:14).

There is no more powerful aid in bearing our mental burdens, than that which comes to us from God, as we pass through the trials and sorrows of this world living with Him.

---

*I used the formula : $\sigma_{P_X} - _{PY} = \sqrt{\dfrac{P_X \, Q_X}{N_X} + \dfrac{P_Y \, Q_Y}{N_Y}}$

Charles C. Peters and Walter R. Van Voorhis, Statistical Procedures and their Mathematical Bases, New York, McGraw-Hill, 1940, p. 183.

[12]Insanity in Priests and Religious. Am. Eccles. Rev., 1936, *95*, p. 487.

INDEX

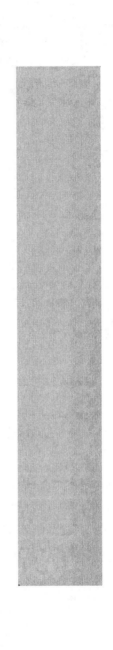

Date Due

APR 29 '61	FE 2 '68	MEt (23622271
	FE 16 '68	Due 4/23/11
MAY 8 '61		
JUN 5 - '61		
AUG 7 '61		
OCT 15 '61		
OCT 30 '61		
NOV 15 '61		
DEC 27 '61		
FEB 26 '62		
MAR 8 - '62		
MAY 25 '62		
AUG 15 '62		
NOV 24 '62		
JA 14 '65		
FE 23 '65		
MY 17 '65		
JA 19 '88		
	PRINTED IN U. S. A.	

CPSIA information can be obtained
at www.ICGtesting.com
Printed in the USA
LVHW082148010722
722611LV00004B/41